Pocket Guide to
Fluid, Electrolyte, and
Acid-Base Balance

Mima M. Horne, R.N., M.S.
Diabetes Nurse Educator
New Hanover Regional Medical Center
Adjunct Faculty
University of North Carolina at Wilmington
Wilmington, North Carolina

Pamela L. Swearingen, R.N.
Special Project Editor
Denver, Colorado

With contributions by:
Ursula Easterday Heitz, R.N., M.S.N.
Nursing Consultant, Nashville, Tennessee

Karen S. Webber, R.N., M.N.
Assistant Professor, School of Nursing
Memorial University of Newfoundland
St. John's, Newfoundland

Second Edition

17 illustrations

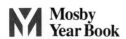

Mosby
Year Book

St. Louis   Baltimore   Boston   Chicago   London   Philadelphia   Sydney   Toronto

Editor: Robin Carter
Production Editor: Victoria Hoenigke
Designer: Jeanne Wolfgeher
Cover Photo: © *Herb Charles Ohlmeyer/Fran Heyl Associates*

M Mosby
Year Book

Dedicated to Publishing Excellence

Second Edition
Copyright © 1993 by Mosby–Year Book, Inc.
A Mosby imprint of Mosby–Year Book, Inc.

Previous edition copyrighted 1989

Printed in the United States of America

Mosby–Year Book, Inc.
11830 Westline Industrial Drive, St. Louis, Missouri 63146

Library of Congress Cataloging in Publication Data
Horne, Mima M.
 Pocket guide to fluid, electrolyte, and acid-base balance / Mima M. Horne, Pamela L. Swearingen, with contributions by Ursula Easterday Heitz and Karen S. Webber. — 2nd ed.
  p. cm.
 Rev. ed. of: Pocket guide to fluids and electrolytes /
[edited by] Mima M. Horne, Pamela L. Swearingen. 1989.
 Includes bibliographical references and index.
 ISBN 0-8016-6689-9 : $18.95
  1. Body fluid disorders — Nursing — Handbooks, manuals, etc.
 2. Water — electrolyte imbalances — Nursing — Handbooks, manuals, etc.
 3. Acid-base imbalances — Nursing — Handbooks, manuals, etc.
 I. Swearingen, Pamela L. II. Pocket guide to fluids and electrolytes.
 III. Title.
  [DNLM: 1. Acid-base imbalance — handbooks. 2. Acid-base Imbalance — nurses' instruction. 3. Body Fluids — handbooks. 4. Body fluids — nurses' instruction. 5. Water-Electrolyte Imbalance — handbooks. 6. Water-Electrolyte Imbalance — nurses' instruction. QU 39 H815p]
RC630.P63   1993
616.3'9 — dc20
DNLM/DLC
for Library of Congress

92-49874
CIP

92 93 94 95 96 CL/DC 9 8 7 6 5 4 3 2 1

Preface

Pocket Guide to Fluid, Electrolyte, and Acid-Base Balance, 2nd edition, was developed to provide nursing students and practicing nurses with quick, practical information on pathophysiology, assessment, diagnostic tests, collaborative management, nursing diagnoses, and nursing interventions for patients with fluid, electrolyte, and acid-base imbalances. Given its portable size, the book is unique in that its coverage of content is both extensive and concise. The organization of the first edition has been retained, with the addition of unit subdivisions to facilitate retrieval of content. Each disorder is presented in a consistent format to enhance utility in the clinical environment. The outline format, boldface headings, use of color, and illustrations reinforce the book's clarity and further enhance its usability. In addition, all efforts have been made to ensure the level of presentation is as easy-to-understand as possible. This is especially important in content related to fluid, electrolyte, and acid-base balance, since the material often is presented in a way that makes comprehension difficult.

Nurses can use this reference for either of two purposes: (1) to identify a patient's specific fluid, electrolyte, or acid-base disturbance and review the nursing diagnoses and care for that specific disturbance; or (2) to identify the medical diagnosis (e.g., diabetic ketoacidosis) and review the discussion of fluid, electrolyte, or acid-base disturbances associated with that particular disorder (i.e., hypokalemia, hypovolemia, hypophosphatemia) and then refer back to the sections that cover these disturbances in detail.

This edition has been thoroughly revised and updated. The pediatrics and geriatrics content has been expanded throughout to address the unique needs of these special patient populations. In addition, the nutrition chapter has been completely updated and expanded to include a discussion of enteral and parenteral nutrition. Acid-base content also has been expanded, including the addition of new tables on interpretation of acid-base imbalance and arterial blood gas results. Although the second edition includes more detailed information about infants and children, the reader is advised that all numbers refer to the adult unless otherwise specified. In addition, the appendices are unusually detailed. They include common abbreviations, a glossary of terms, and normal values for laboratory tests discussed in the text, as well as tables describing the effects of age on fluid, electrolyte, and acid-base balance.

We wish to thank our contributors for a job well done: Ursula Easterday Heitz, who wrote the acid-base section, which comprises Chapters 12–17; and Karen S. Webber, who wrote the nutritional support section. We also thank Melena Segatore, R.N., M.S.N., and Debra Ward, B.Sc., for their editorial assistance in preparation of the nutritional chapter, and the following individuals whose support and suggestions on the first edition were most helpful: Barbara L. Bogdan, R.N., M.S.N., Instructor, South Suburban College of Cook County, South Holland, Illinois; Carol P. Fray, R.N., M.A., Associate Professor, University of North Carolina, Charlotte, North Carolina; and Nancy R. Mitchell, R.N., M.S.N., Instructor, Austin Community College, Riverside Campus, Austin, Texas.

Pocket Guide to Fluid, Electrolyte, and Acid-Base Balance was written to supplement medical-surgical textbooks and assumes the reader has a basic understanding of pathophysiology and assessment. The book also serves as a resource for practicing nurses and academicians. Our primary goals are to make information about fluids, electrolytes, acids, bases, and related topics understandable and to facilitate application of that information to patient care. Reviewers indicate that we have achieved these objectives, and we welcome comments and suggestions from our readers so that we may enhance the book's usefulness in future editions.

Mima M. Horne

Pamela L. Swearingen

Brief Contents

Appendices:

Contents

Unit II Disorders of Fluid, Electrolyte, and Acid-Base Balance 49

6 Disorders of Fluid Balance 51

7 Disorders of Sodium Balance 89

Unit III   Clinical Conditions Associated with Fluid, Electrolyte, and Acid-Base Imbalance   187

Appendices:

BASIC
PRINCIPLES

Overview of Fluid and Electrolyte Balance

The cell is the fundamental functioning unit of the human body. For body cells to perform their individual physiologic tasks, a stable environment is necessary, including maintenance of a steady supply of nutrients and the continuous removal of metabolic wastes. Careful regulation of body fluids helps to ensure a stable internal environment.

Composition of Body Fluids

All body fluids are dilute solutions of water and dissolved substances (solutes).

Water

Water is the major constituent of the human body. The average adult male is approximately 60% water by weight and the average female is approximately 55% water by weight. Factors that affect body water include:

1. **Fat cells:** They contain little water, thus body water decreases with increasing body fat.
2. **Age:** As a rule, body water decreases with increasing age. Premature infants may be as much as 80% water by weight, whereas the full-term infant is approximately 70% water by weight. By the age of 6 months to 1 year, body water decreases to approximately 60%, with little further reduction throughout childhood. The older adult may be 45% to 55% water by weight. See Table 1-1.

Table 1-1   Changes in total body water with age

Age	Kilogram Weight (%)
Premature infant	80
3 mo	70
6 mo	60
1-2 yr	59
11-16 yr	58
Adult	58-60
Obese adult	40-50
Emaciated adult	70-75

From Gröer MW: *Physiology and pathophysiology of the body fluids*, ed 1, St Louis, 1981, Mosby–Year Book.

3. **Female gender:** Women have proportionately less body water due to proportionately greater body fat.

Solutes

In addition to water, body fluids contain two types of dissolved substances (solutes): electrolytes and nonelectrolytes.

1. **Electrolytes:** Substances that dissociate (separate) in solution and will conduct an electrical current. Electrolytes dissociate into positive and negative ions and are measured by their capacity to combine with each other (milliequivalents/liter [mEq/L]) or by their molecular weight in grams (millimoles/liter [mmol/L]). The number of cations and anions, as measured in milliequivalents, in solution is always equal.

   ▪ *Cations:* Ions that develop a positive charge in solution. The primary extracellular cation is sodium (Na^+), whereas the primary intracellular cation is potassium (K^+). A pump system exists in the wall of body cells that pumps sodium out and potassium in.

   ▪ *Anions:* Ions that develop a negative charge in solution. The primary extracellular anion is chloride (Cl^-), whereas the primary intracellular anion is phosphate ion (PO_4^{3-}).

   Because electrolyte content of the plasma and interstitial fluids is essentially the same (see Table 1-2), plasma elec-

Table 1-2 Primary constituents of body fluid compartments

Compartment	Na^+ (mEq/L)	K^+ (mEq/L)	Cl^- (mEq/L)	HCO_3^- (mEq/L)	PO_4^{3-} (mEq/L)
Intravascular (plasma)	142	4.5	104	24	2.0
Interstitial	145	4.4	117	27	2.3
Intracellular (skeletal muscle cell)	12	150	4.0	12	40
Transcellular					
Gastric juice	60	7	100	0	—
Pancreatic juice	130	7	60	100	—
Sweat	45	5	58	0	—

This is a partial list. Other constituents include calcium ion Ca^{2+}, magnesium ion Mg^{2+}, sulfates, proteinates, and organic acids. Note: Values given are average ones. (Modified from Rose BD: Clinical physiology of acid-base and electrolyte disorders, ed 3, New York, 1989, McGraw-Hill Co.)

trolyte values reflect the composition of the extracellular fluid, which is composed of intravascular and interstitial fluids (see below). However, plasma electrolyte values do not necessarily reflect the electrolyte composition of the intracellular fluid. Understanding the difference between these two compartments is important in anticipating the types of imbalances that can occur with certain disorders such as tissue trauma or acid-base imbalances. In these situations, electrolytes may be released from or move into or out of the cells, significantly altering plasma electrolyte values. See discussions of potassium balance, p. 97, and phosphorus balance, p. 118.

2. **Nonelectrolytes:** Substances such as glucose and urea that do not dissociate in solution and are measured by weight (milligrams per 100 ml — mg/dl). Other clinically important nonelectrolytes include *creatinine* and *bilirubin*.

Fluid Compartments

Body fluids are distributed between two major fluid compartments: the intracellular compartment and the extracellular compartment (Figure 1-1).

Intracellular Fluid (ICF)

ICF is the fluid contained within the cells. In the adult, approximately two thirds of the body's fluid is intracellular, equalling approximately 25 L in the average (70 kg) adult male. In contrast, only half of an infant's body fluid is intracellular.

Extracellular Fluid (ECF)

ECF is the fluid outside the cells. The *relative* size of ECF decreases with advancing age. In the newborn, approximately half the body fluid is contained within ECF. After the age of one year, the *relative* volume of ECF decreases to approximately one third of the total volume. This equals approximately 15 L in the average (70 kg) adult male. ECF is further divided into the following:

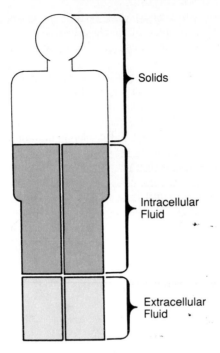

Figure 1-1.   Comparison of intracellular fluid to extracellular fluid.

1. **Interstitial fluid (ISF):** The fluid surrounding the cells, equal to approximately 8 L in the adult. Lymph fluid is included in the interstitial volume. Relative to body size, the volume of ISF is approximately twice as great in the newborn as in the adult.

2. **Intravascular fluid (IVF):** The fluid contained within the blood vessels. The *relative* volume of IVF is similar in adults and children. Average adult blood volume is approximately 5-6 L, of which about 3 L is plasma. The remaining 2-3 L consist of red blood cells (RBCs, or erythrocytes) which transport oxygen and act as important body

buffers; white blood cells (WBCs, or leukocytes); and platelets. Functions of the blood include:
- Delivery of nutrients (e.g., glucose and oxygen) to the tissues.
- Transport of waste products to the kidneys and lungs.
- Delivery of antibodies and WBCs to sites of infection.
- Transport of hormones to their sites of action.
- Circulation of body heat.

3. **Transcellular fluid (TCF):** The fluid contained within specialized cavities of the body. Examples of TCF include cerebrospinal, pericardial, pleural, synovial, and intraocular fluids, and digestive secretions. At any given time, TCF is approximately 1 L. However, large amounts of fluid may move into and out of the transcellular space each day. For example, the gastrointestinal (GI) tract normally secretes and reabsorbs up to 6-8 L per day.

Factors that Affect Movement of Water and Solutes

Membranes

Each of the fluid compartments is separated by a selectively permeable membrane that permits the movement of water and some solutes. Although small molecules such as urea and water move freely between all compartments, certain substances move less readily. Plasma proteins, for example, are restricted to the IVF owing to the low permeability of the capillary membrane to large molecules. Selective permeability of membranes helps to maintain the unique composition of each compartment while allowing for the movement of nutrients from the plasma to the cells and the movement of waste products out of the cells and eventually into the plasma. The body's semipermeable membranes include:

1. **Cell membranes:** Separate ICF from ISF and are composed of lipids and protein.
2. **Capillary membranes:** Separate IVF from ISF.
3. **Epithelial membranes:** Separate ISF and IVF from TCF. Examples of epithelial membranes include the mucosal epithelium of the stomach and intestines, the synovial membrane, and the renal tubules.

Transport Processes

In addition to membrane selectivity, the movement of water and solutes is determined by several transport processes.

1. **Diffusion:** The random movement of particles in all directions through a solution or gas. Particles move from an area of high concentration to an area of low concentration along a concentration gradient. The energy for diffusion is produced by thermal energy. An example of diffusion is the movement of oxygen from the alveoli of the lung to the blood of the pulmonary capillaries. Diffusion also may occur because of changes in electrical potential across the membrane. Cations will follow anions and vice versa. See Table 1-3 for a list of factors that increase diffusion (opposite factors will act to reduce diffusion).

   Cell walls are composed of sheets of lipids with many minute protein pores. Substances may diffuse across the cell wall under the following conditions:

   - If they are small enough to pass through the protein pores (e.g., water and urea): This is termed *simple diffusion.*
   - If they are lipid soluble (e.g., oxygen and carbon dioxide): This is another example of simple diffusion.
   - By means of a carrier substance: This is termed *facilitated diffusion.* Large lipid-insoluble substance such as glucose must diffuse into the cell *via* a carrier substance. Glucose, for example, combines with a carrier on the outside of the cell to become lipid soluble. Once inside the cell, glucose breaks away from the carrier and the carrier is then free to facilitate diffusion of additional glucose.

Table 1-3   Factors that increase diffusion*

- Increased temperature
- Increased concentration of the particle
- Decreased size or molecular weight of the particle
- Increased surface area available for diffusion
- Decreased distance across which the particle mass must diffuse

---

*Note: Opposite factors will act to reduce diffusion.

As with simple diffusion, facilitated diffusion requires the presence of a concentration gradient that favors diffusion. The rate of facilitated diffusion, however, depends on the availability of the carrier substance. If there is a large concentration gradient (i.e., the difference between the areas of high and low concentration is great), the carrier can become saturated (used up) and diffusion will decrease despite the presence of a favorable concentration gradient. Glucose will move into the cell, for example, only if there is a favorable concentration gradient and an available carrier substance.

2. **Active transport:** Simple diffusion will not occur in the absence of a favorable electrical or concentration gradient. Energy is required for a substance to move from an area of lesser or equal concentration to an area of equal or higher concentration. This is termed *active transport,* and like facilitated diffusion, it depends on the availability of carrier substances. Many important solutes are transported actively across cell membranes, including sodium, potassium, hydrogen, glucose, and amino acids. The renal tubules, for example, depend on active transport to reabsorb all the glucose filtered by the glomeruli to enable excretion of urine that is glucose-free. As with facilitated diffusion, the carriers can become overwhelmed or saturated. In the case of glucose within the renal tubule, saturation occurs when the blood sugar exceeds approximately 180-200 mg/dl. Active transport is vital for maintaining the unique composition of both the ECF and ICF.

3. **Filtration:** The movement of water and solutes from an area of high hydrostatic pressure to an area of low hydrostatic pressure. *Hydrostatic pressure* is the pressure created by the weight of fluid. Filtration is important in directing fluid out of the arterial end of the capillaries. It is also the force that enables the kidneys to filter 180 L of plasma per day.

4. **Osmosis:** The movement of water across a semipermeable membrane from an area of lower solute concentration to an area of higher solute concentration. Osmosis can occur across any membrane when solute concentrations on either side of the membrane change. The following are terms that are associated with osmosis:

- *Osmotic pressure:* The amount of hydrostatic pressure required to stop the osmotic flow of water.
- *Oncotic pressure:* The osmotic pressure exerted by colloids (proteins). Albumin, for example, exerts oncotic pressure within the blood vessels and helps hold the water content of the blood in the intravascular space.
- *Osmotic diuresis:* Increased urine output caused by substances such as mannitol, glucose, or contrast media, which are excreted in the urine and reduce renal water reabsorption. An osmotic diuresis occurs in uncontrolled diabetes mellitus, for example, due to the presence of excess glucose in the renal tubule. When the blood sugar is within normal range, all the glucose that is filtered by the kidney is reabsorbed (saved) *via* active transport. In hyperglycemia (blood sugar >180-200 mg/dl), the kidney's ability to reabsorb glucose is overwhelmed (i.e., the carrier substance becomes saturated). The glucose that is not reabsorbed remains in the tubule and acts osmotically to hold water that otherwise would be reabsorbed. The net result is *glucosuria* and *polyuria.*

Concentration of Body Fluids

1. **Osmolality:** As discussed above, changes in the concentration of body fluids affect the movement of water between fluid compartments by osmosis. The measure of a solution's ability to create osmotic pressure and thus affect the movement of water is termed *osmolality*. Osmolality also may be described as a measure of the concentration of body fluids (the ratio of solutes to water) because it is reported in milliosmoles (1 one thousandth of an osmole) per kilogram of water (mOsm/kg). One osmole contains 6×10^{23} particles. *Osmolarity,* another term used to describe the concentration of solutions, reflects the number of particles in a liter of solution and is measured in milliosmoles per liter (mOsm/L). Because body fluids are relatively dilute, the difference between their osmolality and osmolarity is small, and the terms often are used interchangeably. Osmolality is the measure used to evaluate serum and urine in clinical practice.

   Changes in extracellular osmolality may result in

changes in both extracellular and intracellular fluid volume:

Decreased ECF osmolality → *movement of water from the ECF to the ICF*

Increased ECF osmolality → *movement of water from the ICF to the ECF*

Water will continue to move until the osmolality of the two compartments reaches equilibrium. This is the rationale for using intravenous (IV) mannitol in the treatment of cerebral edema. Mannitol increases the osmolality of the ECF, promoting the movement of water out of the cerebral cells, thereby reducing cellular swelling.

Osmolality of the ECF may be determined by measuring serum osmolality (see Chapter 5 for additional information). Sodium is the primary determinant of ECF osmolality. Because it is limited primarily to the ECF, sodium acts to hold water in that compartment. Potassium helps to maintain the volume of ICF, and the plasma proteins help to maintain the volume of the intravascular space (IVS).

2. **Tonicity:** Small molecules like urea that readily cross all membranes quickly equilibrate between compartments and have little effect on the movement of water. These small molecules are termed *ineffective osmoles.* In contrast, sodium, glucose, and mannitol are examples of *effective osmoles;* they do not cross the cell membrane quickly and will, therefore, affect the movement of water. Thus *effective osmolality* (i.e., osmolality that will cause water to move from one compartment to another) is dependent not only on the number of solutes, but also on the permeability of the membrane to these solutes. *Tonicity* is another term for effective osmolality.

- *Isotonic solutions:* Those that have the same effective osmolality as body fluids (approximately 280-300 mOsm/kg). An example is normal saline—0.9% sodium chloride (NaCl) solution.

- *Hypotonic solutions:* Those that have an effective osmolality less than body fluids. An example is 0.45% NaCl solution.

- *Hypertonic solutions:* Those that have an effective osmolality greater than body fluids. An example is 3% NaCl solution.

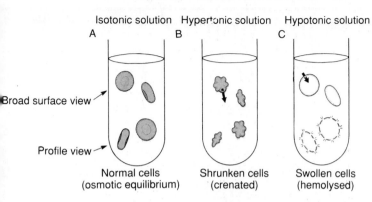

Figure 1-2.   Effect of osmotic pressure on the cells.

Clinical hypotonicity occurs when there is an abnormal gain in water or loss of sodium-rich fluids with replacement by water only. *Clinical hypertonicity* may develop owing to loss of water (e.g., diabetes insipidus), loss of hypotonic body fluids (e.g., sweating, diarrhea), or gain of effective osmoles (e.g., hyperglycemia or administration of hypertonic NaCl, sodium bicarbonate [$NaHCO_3$], or mannitol). Hyperosmolality *without* hypertonicity (does not cause cellular dehydration) occurs in renal failure due to retention of urea. See Figure 1-2 for a depiction of osmotic pressure on the cells.

Regulation of Vascular Volume and Extracellular Fluid (ECF) Osmolality

2

To provide an optimal environment for the body's cells, the composition, concentration, and volume of the ECF are regulated by a combination of renal, metabolic, and neurologic functions. The ECF is continuously altered and then modified as the body reacts with its surrounding environment. In contrast, the intracellular fluid (ICF) is protected by the ECF and remains relatively stable, ensuring normal cellular function. Because the primary constituents of the ECF are water and sodium (and sodium's accompanying anions), their regulation is crucial for maintaining the volume and concentration of the ECF (Figures 2-1, 2-2, and 2-3). Regulation of the composition of the ECF depends on the regulation of the individual electrolytes (see Chapters 7 through 11).

Regulation of Vascular Volume

Large fluctuations can occur in the volume of the interstitial portion of the ECF without markedly affecting body functions. This is especially true if the changes occur slowly. Individuals with cirrhosis, for example, often are able to tolerate significant amounts of ascitic fluid. The vascular portion of the ECF is less tolerant of change and must be maintained carefully to ensure

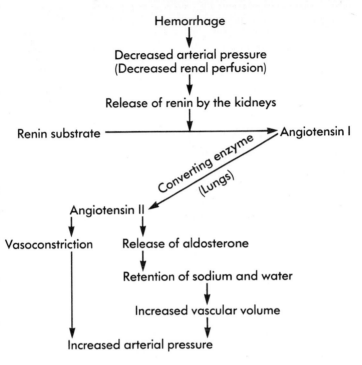

Figure 2-1. Action of the renin-angiotensin-aldosterone system: a clinical example.

that the tissues receive an adequate supply of nutrients and continuous removal of metabolic wastes without compromising the cardiovascular system. The portion of the intravascular fluid (IVF) that effectively perfuses tissues is termed the effective circulating volume (ECV).

Changes in the ECV are sensed by specialized receptors located in the carotid sinuses, aortic arch, cardiac artria, and renal vessels. These volume receptors do not measure total volume but rather, respond to changes in pressure *via* changes in stretch in the arterial or atrial wall. Increases in ECV cause an increase in blood pressure and thus stretch at these receptors. In contrast, a decrease in ECV causes a decrease in pressure and stretch. Changes in volume sensed by the volume receptors lead to

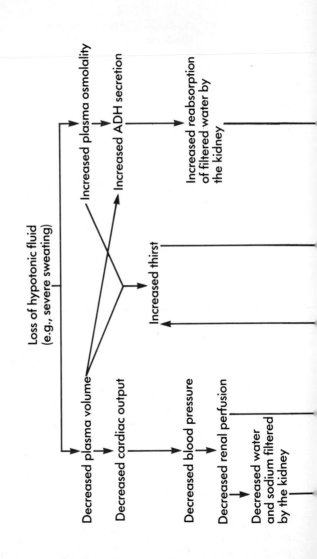

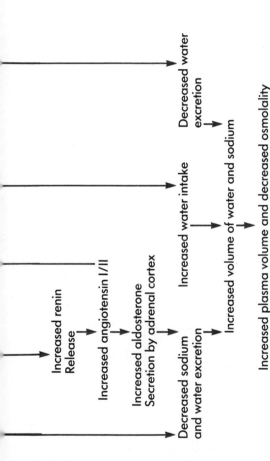

Increased renin Release

Increased angiotensin I/II

Increased aldosterone Secretion by adrenal cortex

Decreased sodium and water excretion

Increased volume of water and sodium

Increased water intake

Decreased water excretion

Increased plasma volume and decreased osmolality

Figure 2-2. Regulation of fluid volume and osmolality: a clinical example.

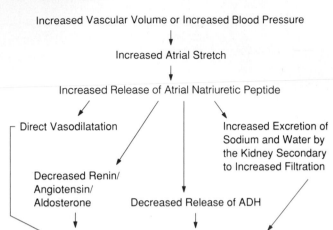

Figure 2-3. Action of the atrial natriuretic peptide in reducing vascular volume or blood pressure.

changes in cardiac output, vascular resistance, thirst, and renal handling of sodium and water. These changes are mediated by a combination of interrelated neurologic and hormonal functions described in subsequent sections.

Sympathetic Nervous System

The sympathetic nervous system provides the initial compensatory response to rapid or short-term changes in the ECV. Changes in stretch sensed by the volume receptors lead to changes in sympathetic tone. Decreased ECV, for example, results in increased sympathetic tone. Increased sympathetic tone causes the following:

1. **Increased cardiac output:** Secondary to an increase in cardiac contractility, conduction, and rate.
2. **Increased arterial resistance.**
3. **Increased release of renin by the kidneys:** Leads to an increase in the release of aldosterone by the adrenal cortex (see Figure 2-1).

Items 1 and 2 act to raise blood pressure only. Item 3 leads to both an increase in blood pressure and an increase in vascular volume owing to the retention of sodium and water.

Renin-Angiotensin

Renin is a proteolytic enzyme produced and released by the kidney in response to decreased renal perfusion (secondary to a reduction in ECV) or increased sympathetic nervous system stimulation. Renin acts on angiotensinogen to produce angiotensin I, which is converted to angiotensin II, a potent vasoconstrictor. Angiotensin II, in turn, stimulates the release of aldosterone. Certain antihypertensive medications (e.g., captopril) act in part by preventing the conversion of angiotensin I to angiotensin II.

Aldosterone

Renin also raises blood pressure through the actions of aldosterone. Aldosterone is a mineralcorticoid hormone released by the adrenal cortex, which acts on the distal portion of the renal tubule to increase the reabsorption (saving) of sodium and the secretion and excretion of potassium and hydrogen. Because sodium retention leads to water retention, aldosterone acts as a volume regulator. Factors that increase the release of aldosterone include the following:

1. **Increased renin levels.**
2. **Increased plasma potassium levels.**
3. **Decreased plasma sodium levels.**
4. **Increased ACTH levels.**

Atrial Natriuretic Peptide (ANP)

ANP, also known as atrial natriuretic factor, is a recently identified hormone released by the cardiac atria in response to increased atrial pressure. In contrast to the renin-angiotensin-aldosterone system, ANP acts to reduce blood pressure and vascular volume. Its actions include the following:

1. **Increased excretion of sodium and water by the kidney** secondary to increased filtration.
2. **Decreased synthesis of renin and decreased release of aldosterone.**

3. **Decreased release of antidiuretic hormone (ADH).**
4. **Direct vasodilatation.**

ANP is released in response to any condition that causes volume expansion, or elevated cardiac filling pressures, e.g., congestive heart failure (CHF), chronic renal failure, use of vasoconstrictor agents, and atrial tachycardia (see Figure 2-3). If analogs (man-made substances with similar structure and function) of ANP can be developed, potentially they may be useful in the management of hypertension, congestive heart failure, renal failure, and other volume overload states.

Antidiuretic Hormone (ADH) and Thirst

Both ADH and thirst assist in the regulation of vascular volume. For a discussion of their actions see below.

Regulation of Extracellular Fluid (ECF) Osmolality

The osmolality or concentration of the ECF will determine whether fluid moves into or out of the cells.

Increased ECF osmolality → cells shrivel
Decreased ECF osmolality → cells swell

Thus it is critical that the ECF osmolality be maintained within a narrow range to protect cellular function. The primary symptoms of altered plasma osmolality are neurologic (e.g., irritability, personality changes, seizures, coma) and reflect the changes in brain cell function.

Because sodium is the primary solute of the ECF, it is also the primary determinant of ECF osmolality. Two control systems work together to maintain the sodium/water ratio: ADH and thirst.

Antidiuretic Hormone (ADH)

ADH is a hormone produced by the hypothalamus and secreted into the general circulation by the posterior pituitary gland. It acts on the collecting duct in the kidney to increase the reabsorption (saving) of water and allow the excretion of a concentrated urine. Factors that increase the release of ADH are found in Ta-

Table 2-1   Factors that increase the release of ADH*

- Increased plasma osmolality sensed by osmoreceptors located within the hypothalamus.
- Decreased ECV sensed by volume receptors located within the pulmonary vasculature and the left atria.
- Decreased blood pressure sensed by baroreceptors.
- Stress and pain.
- Medications, including morphine and barbiturates.
- Surgery and certain anesthetics.
- Positive pressure ventilators.

*See Chapter 20 for a discussion of disorders that lead to inappropriate or excessive production of ADH.

Table 2-2   Factors that decrease the release of ADH*

- Decreased plasma osmolality.
- Increased ECV.
- Increased blood pressure.
- Medications, including phenytoin and ethyl alcohol.

*See Chapter 20 for a discussion of disorders that lead to a reduction in ADH activity or release.

Table 2-3   Medications that alter the action of ADH

Suppress	Enhance
Lithium	Chlorpropamide
Demeclocycline	Indomethacin
Methoxyflurane	

ble 2-1; factors that decrease the release of ADH are found in Table 2-2. ADH also is an arterial vasoconstrictor that acts to raise blood pressure by increasing vascular resistance. ADH is regulated primarily by changes in plasma osmolality and effective circulating volume. Additional factors that affect the release of ADH are emotions and medications (see Chapter 20).

In addition to medications that affect the release of ADH, there are also medications that suppress or enhance the action of ADH on the renal collecting duct (Table 2-3).

Thirst

In addition to ADH, thirst also acts to regulate the ECF concentration and is stimulated by essentially the same factors that increase the release of ADH: increased plasma osmolality, volume depletion, and hypotension. Increased angiotensin II levels and dry mucous membranes (the sensation of a dry mouth) also stimulate thirst. Thirst is not as carefully regulated as ADH because it is affected strongly by social and emotional factors. However, thirst does provide the primary protection against hyperosmolality. Symptomatic hyperosmolality occurs only in individuals who do not have a normal thirst mechanism or who do not have access to water. Thus, hyperosmolality typically occurs in infants or comatose patients who are unable to ask for water. Alert patients with diabetes insipidus, for example, who excrete a large, abnormally dilute urine due to altered ADH function, will maintain a relatively normal osmolality and volume as long as they are able to drink and satisfy their thirst.

Fluid Gains
and Losses

3

In health there is a steady state or balance between the fluids gained and lost by the body. As discussed in Chapter 2, the volume, concentration, and composition of body fluids are regulated so that output matches intake and balance is maintained. Loss of hypotonic fluids, for example, leads to decreased water excretion and increased thirst. This physiologic balance is termed *homeostasis*. This chapter reviews the means of normal and abnormal fluid gains and losses. Table 3-1 lists daily fluid gains and losses in approximate amounts.

Fluid Gains
Oxidative Metabolism

Approximately 300 ml of water are produced daily by the oxidation of carbohydrates, proteins, and fat. That is, oxygen combines with some of the hydrogen in these substances to produce water. This amount of water is insufficient to compensate for the body's obligatory fluid losses, thus some additional oral, parenteral, or enteral intake is necessary to maintain body vol-

Table 3-1   Average daily fluid gains and losses in the adult

Fluid Gains		Fluid Losses	
Oxidative metabolism	300 ml	Kidneys	1200-1500 ml
Oral fluids	1100-1400 ml	Skin	500-600 ml
Solid foods	800-1000 ml	Lungs	400 ml
Total	2200-2700 ml	GI	100-200 ml
		Total	2200-2700 ml

ume. Under the best of conditions, individuals may survive weeks without food intake but only days without water intake.

Oral Fluids

Approximately 1100-1400 ml of fluid are consumed orally per day. Fluid intake varies greatly as thirst is not accurately regulated in humans and is affected by social and emotional, as well as physiologic factors (see Chapter 2, p. 22).

Solid Food

Fluid is gained through the consumption of solid food, which provides approximately 800-1000 ml of water each day. Meat, for example, is approximately 70% water, and fruits and vegetables are over 90% water by weight.

Fluid Therapy

Fluid also may be gained through parenteral or enteral routes and by means of irrigants that are retained. If a nasogastric (NG) tube is irrigated, for example, and an equal amount is not withdrawn and discarded, the extra irrigant must be considered a fluid gain. Mechanical ventilation with humidified gases may result in a net gain of water by the lungs. See Chapter 6 for a discussion of parenteral fluid therapy and Chapter 26 for a discussion of all types of nutritional therapy.

Fluid Losses
Kidneys

The kidneys are the primary regulators of fluid and electrolyte balance. Approximately 180 L of plasma are filtered daily by the kidneys. From this volume, approximately 1500 ml of urine are excreted each day. Hourly urine output has an *average range* of 40-80 ml for adults and 0.5 mL/kg/hr for children. The volume, composition, and concentration of urine varies greatly and will depend on intake and other fluid losses. Urine values (volume and concentration) always should be evaluated in relation to the body's need to conserve or excrete fluid. The dehydrated patient who needs to conserve fluid, for example, would be expected to excrete less urine than the patient who is adequately hydrated.

The concentration of urine may range from 50 to 1400 mOsm/kg. Although sodium is the primary determinant of extracellular fluid (ECF) osmolality or concentration, metabolic wastes are the primary determinant of urinary osmolality or concentration. Therefore, in severe hypovolemia or hypotension, for example, the kidneys are able to excrete a concentrated yet relatively sodium-free urine.

1. **Normal urinary output:** At maximal urinary concentration (1400 mOsm/kg), at least 400 ml of urine must be produced to excrete the daily load of metabolic wastes. Infants, the elderly, and individuals with renal disease who cannot maximally concentrate their urine will have greater obligatory water losses. That is, they will need to produce a proportionately larger volume of urine in order to excrete their daily load of metabolic wastes. Average daily urine output is 1500 ml.

2. **Oliguria:** Urinary output of less than 400 ml/24 hr. It signals the retention of metabolic wastes.

3. **Anuria:** Production of less than 100 ml of urine in 24 hr.

4. **Polyuria:** An abnormally large amount of urinary output.

Skin

An average of 500-600 ml of sensible and insensible fluid are lost *via* the skin each day.

1. **Insensible fluid:** Loss is evaporative from the skin and occurs without the individual's awareness. It is lost at a rate of 6 ml/kg/24 hr in the average adult, but can increase significantly with fever or burns. Low-birthweight infants, especially those weighing less than 1 kg, are prone to extremely high rates of insensible fluid loss owing to multiple factors, including larger skin surface area and increased skin water content. Use of radiant warmers will significantly increase insensible fluid loss in the neonate. Insensible fluid is nearly electrolyte-free and should be considered pure water loss.

2. **Sensible fluid (i.e., sweat):** Important in dissipating body heat, and like insensible fluid, it is hypotonic. Sensible fluid, however, does contain a significant amount of elec-

trolytes (see Table 1-2, p. 5). The rate of sensible fluid loss varies greatly with the individual's activity level and the ambient temperature. In extreme cases, sensible fluid loss may be as great as 2 L/hr.

Lungs

Approximately 400 ml of insensible fluid are lost through the lungs each day. This amount may increase with increased respiratory depth or dry climate.

Gastrointestinal (GI) Tract

Under normal conditions, the GI tract accounts for only 100-200 ml fluid loss each day, yet it plays a vital role in fluid regulation because it is the site of nearly all fluid gain. In disease, however, the GI tract may become a site of major fluid loss, because approximately 6-8 L of isotonic fluid are secreted into and reabsorbed out of the GI tract daily. This is equal to approximately half the ECF volume. Thus, abnormal GI losses (e.g., NG suction, vomiting, diarrhea) may lead to profound fluid loss. The composition of the GI secretions varies with the location within the GI tract. Above the pylorus, the losses are isotonic and rich in sodium, potassium, chloride, and hydrogen. Below the pylorus, losses are isotonic and rich in sodium, potassium, and bicarbonate (see Table 1-2, p. 5). Diarrhea from the large intestine is hypotonic. See Chapter 18 for additional information.

Additional Losses

Significant amounts of fluid may be lost due to increased evaporative loss from large open wounds, draining wounds, fistulas, or external bleeding. Crying may contribute significantly to fluid loss in small children.

Third-Space Losses

The loss of ECF into a normally nonequilibrating space is termed *third-space fluid shift*. Although this fluid is not lost from the body, it is temporarily unavailable for use by either the intracellular fluid (ICF) or ECF. Third-space fluid losses must be considered when evaluating the adequacy of fluid therapy. See Table 6-1 for a list of disorders associated with third-space fluid shifts.

Nursing Assessment of the Patient at Risk

4

Fluid and electrolyte homeostasis is essential for health and well being. Unfortunately, fluid, electrolyte, and acid-base disturbances are potential complications of almost all disease states and medical therapies. Nurses in all areas of practice must be diligent in their assessment of individuals at risk for developing fluid, electrolyte, and acid-base disturbances.

Nursing History

Each of the following dimensions of the health history should be considered.

Physiologic

1. Does the individual have any disease or disorders that may cause a disturbance in fluid and electrolyte homeostasis (e.g., ulcerative colitis, diabetes mellitus)?
2. Is the individual receiving any medications or therapy that may cause a disturbance in fluid, electrolyte, and acid-base status (e.g., diuretics, nasogastric suction)?

Developmental

Is the individual at increased risk because of age or social situation (e.g., an elderly adult who lives alone)? **Note:** Fluid volume deficit is more common in infants and the elderly. (See Appendix E.)

Psychologic

Are there behavioral or emotional problems that may increase the risk of fluid, electrolyte, and acid-base disturbances (e.g., denial and noncompliance with a medical regimen in a diabetic teenager)?

Spiritual

Does the individual have any beliefs, values, or practices that may affect his or her ability to comply with medical interventions (e.g., the Jehovah's Witness with GI bleeding who refuses human blood products)?

Sociocultural

Are there any social, cultural, financial, or educational factors that place the individual at increased risk or affect his or her ability to comply with medical therapy (e.g., the patient on a fixed income who, in an attempt to save money, fills only the digoxin and diuretic prescriptions, but not the potassium supplement prescription)?

Clinical Assessment

Two of the most important tools for the clinical assessment of fluid balance problems are simple nursing procedures that may be initiated without a physician's order: daily weights and intake and output. Hemodynamic monitoring is an invasive means of assessing fluid balance disorders.

Daily Weights

Acute weight changes are usually indicative of *acute* fluid changes. Each kilogram of weight lost or gained suggests one liter of fluid lost or gained. Thus, a 2-kg acute weight loss equals a 2-L fluid loss. Weight gains do not necessarily indicate an increase in effective circulating volume, but rather, an increase in total body volume that may be located in any of the fluid compartments. For accuracy and consistency, weight should be measured at the same time of day, preferably before breakfast. The scale should be balanced before each use and the individual should be weighed wearing approximately the same clothing. The type of scale (i.e., standing, bed, chair) should be noted so that whenever possible the same scale can be used.

Intake and Output (I&O)

All I&O should be accurately measured whenever possible and all unmeasured volumes estimated and noted. The I&O record should include the following:

1. **Intake:**
   - *Oral fluids:* Ice chips must be included and recorded as fluids at approximately one half their volume. Include all foods that are liquid at room temperature.
   - *Parenteral fluids:* Parenteral fluid containers are often overfilled and the excess should be discarded during setup or the exact amount given recorded.
   - *Tube feedings:* Often a 30-50 ml water flush is given at the end of intermittent tube feedings or periodically during continuous tube feedings. This flush needs to be included in the intake record.
   - *Catheter irrigants:* If the catheter is irrigated or lavaged and an equal amount is not withdrawn and discarded, the extra irrigant should be added to the intake record.
2. **Output:**
   - *Urine output:* Ideally, it is measured hourly.
   - *Liquid feces.*
   - *Vomitus.*
   - *NG drainage.*
   - *Excessive sweating:* May be documented either *via* a rating system (1+ for noticeable sweating to 4+ for profuse sweating) or by documenting the amount of linen saturated with sweat.
   - *Wound drainage:* May be documented by noting the type and number of dressings saturated, by weighing dressings, or by direct measurement of drainage contained in a gravity or vacuum drainage device (e.g., Hemovac, drainage bags).
   - *Draining fistulas:* If possible, collect drainage in a stoma bag or document amount of dressings or linen saturated.

- *Rapid or labored respiratory rate:* Will contribute to a patient's insensible fluid loss and should be documented.

Hemodynamic Monitoring

Hemodynamic monitoring may be useful in evaluating fluid volume abnormalities. See Table 4-1, below.

1. **Central venous pressure (CVP):** Measures mean right atrial pressure and right ventricular end-diastolic pressure by means of a catheter that is inserted in or near the right atrium. A normal reading is 2-6 mm Hg or 5-12 cm H_2O.

2. **Pulmonary artery pressure (PAP):** Measured by means of a catheter passed through the right heart and into the pulmonary artery (PA) with the tip positioned in the pulmonary capillary bed. Normal PAP is 20-30/8-15 mm Hg. PA diastolic pressures may be used to estimate left ventricular end-diastolic pressure and thus evaluate cardiac performance.

Table 4-1 Hemodynamic evaluation of fluid volume abnormalities

Clinical Reading	Potential Cause
CVP < 2 mm Hg or <5 cm H_2O PAP < 20/8 mm Hg	Decreased effective circulating volume owing to true volume depletion (e.g., bleeding), shifting of fluid out of the vascular space (e.g., burns), or vasodilatation (e.g., after administration of certain antihypertensive medications).
CVP > 6 mm Hg or > 12 cm H_2O	Fluid overload, poor right ventricular function, or constriction of the pulmonary vascular bed.
PAP > 30/15 mm Hg	Increases in fluid volume or in pulmonary vascular resistance.

Vital Signs

The following are examples of changes in vital signs that may signal fluid, electrolyte, or acid-base imbalance.

Body Temperature

1. **Elevations in body temperature:** May lead to fluid and electrolyte losses due to increased insensible loss. Hypernatremic (elevated sodium) dehydration may cause an elevation in temperature.
2. **Decreases in body temperature:** May result from hypovolemia. In severe fluid volume deficit, the rectal temperature may drop to as low as 35°C (95°F).

Respiratory Rate and Depth

1. **Increases in respiratory rate and depth:** Increase insensible fluid loss and may contribute to the development of volume depletion.
2. **Rapid, deep respirations:** May be compensation for metabolic acidosis.
3. **Shortness of breath (SOB), crackles (rales), or rhonchi:** May signal fluid buildup in the lungs due to fluid volume excess.

Heart Rate/Pulses

1. **Heart rate:** Increased heart rate may occur with fluid volume deficit as a compensatory mechanism for maintaining cardiac output.
2. **Bounding pulse:** May signal fluid volume excess. The strength and volume of the pulse is dependent on the volume of blood ejected by the left ventricle and the strength of the left ventricular contraction. Both may increase in fluid volume excess.
3. **Weak, thready pulse:** May signal fluid volume deficit due to a reduction in intravascular volume.
4. **Irregular heart rate:** May occur with hypokalemia or hypomagnesemia secondary to the development of dysrhythmias.

Blood Pressure (BP)

Blood pressure is determined by multiplying cardiac output (CO) by systemic vascular resistance (SVR). Cardiac output, in turn, is the product of heart rate multiplied by stroke volume (the amount of blood moved with each contraction of the left ventricle). Thus, changes in stroke volume, heart rate, or vascular resistance may result in changes in blood pressure.

1. **Decreased BP:** May signal fluid volume deficit owing to a reduction in stroke volume. Electrolyte imbalances that cause dysrhythmias may decrease BP if either heart rate or stroke volume is affected.
2. **Elevated BP:** May signal fluid volume excess because of an increase in stroke volume.

Physical Assessment

The following are some examples of changes noted on physical assessment that may be indicative of fluid, electrolyte, or acid-base imbalance. See individual fluid and electrolyte disorders, Chapters 6 through 11, and the acid-base disorders, Chapters 12 through 17, for additional information.

Integument

1. **Flushed, dry skin:** May signal fluid volume deficit.
2. **Changes in skin turgor:** May reflect changes in interstitial fluid volume. Turgor may be assessed by pinching skin over the forearm, sternum, or dorsum of the hand. With adequate hydration, the pinched skin returns quickly to its original position when released. With fluid volume deficit, the pinched skin stays elevated for several seconds. This is a less reliable indicator in the elderly owing to the skin's decreased elasticity.
3. **Edema:** Indicates an expanded interstitial volume. It may be localized (usually the result of inflammation) or generalized (due to altered capillary hemodynamics and the retention of excess sodium and water) and usually is most evident in dependent areas. The presence of periorbital edema suggests significant fluid retention. Pitting should be assessed over a bony surface such as the tibia or sacrum

and rated according to severity (i.e., 1+ for barely detect-
able edema to 4+ for deep, persistent pitting [see Figure
6-3]). See Chapter 6 for additional information.
4. **Increased furrowing of the tongue:** Suggestive of fluid
volume deficit.
5. **Decreased moisture between the cheek and gum in the
oral cavity:** Signals fluid volume deficit.

Cardiovascular System

1. **Assessment of jugular venous distention:** Provides an estimate of central venous pressure. With the head of bed
(HOB) at a 30- to 45-degree angle, measure the distance
between the level of the sternal angle (Angle of Louis) and
the point at which the internal and external jugular veins
collapse. Optimally this distance should be 3 cm or less
(Figure 4-1). Values of greater than 3 cm suggest fluid
volume excess or decreased cardiac function.
2. **Assessment of the veins of the hands:** May be used to assess fluid volume status. Normally, elevating the hand will
collapse the veins in 3-5 seconds and lowering the hand
will refill them in 3-5 seconds. With fluid volume deficit,
the veins of the lowered hand require more than 3-5 seconds to fill. With fluid volume excess, the veins of the elevated hand require more than 3-5 seconds to empty.
3. **Dysrhythmias:** May occur with potassium, calcium, and
magnesium abnormalities (see individual sections for a
discussion of specific electrocardiogram [ECG] changes).

Neurologic System

1. **Changes in level of consciousness (LOC):** Occur with
changes in serum osmolality or changes in serum sodium.
The severity of the symptoms will depend on the rate and
degree of change. Changes in LOC also may occur with
acute acid-base imbalances.
2. **Restlessness and confusion:** May occur with fluid volume
deficit or acid-base imbalance.
3. **Abnormal reflexes:** Occur with calcium and magnesium
changes. Calcium and magnesium deficits enhance neuro-

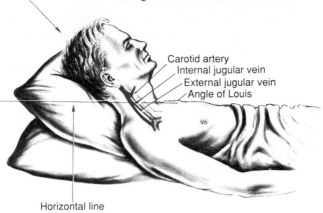

Carotid artery
Internal jugular vein
External jugular vein
Angle of Louis

Horizontal line

Figure 4-1.   Inspection of external jugular venous pressure.
From Thompson J, et al. Clinical nursing, ed 2, St Louis, 1990,
Mosby–Year Book.

muscular excitability (e.g., hyperactive reflexes), whereas
calcium and magnesium excesses depress neuromuscular
function (e.g., diminished reflexes).

4. **Positive Trousseau's sign and Chvostek's sign:** Can oc-
   cur with hypocalcemia and hypomagnesemia.
   - *Positive Trousseau's sign:* Ischemia-induced carpal
     spasm. It is elicited by applying a BP cuff to the upper
     arm and inflating it past systolic BP for 2 minutes.
   - *Positive Chvostek's sign:* Unilateral contraction of the
     facial and eyelid muscles. It is elicited when irritating
     the facial nerve by percussing the face just in front of
     the ear.

5. **Neuromuscular changes resulting from altered membrane polarization of excitable tissue:** Caused by abnormalities in potassium or calcium levels. For example, neuromuscular symptoms of tingling, paresthesias, weakness,
   and flaccid paralysis may occur with hyperkalemia. Weakness, cramps, dysrhythmias, and paralysis may occur with
   hypokalemia. Neuromuscular irritability and paresthesias
   also may occur with metabolic alkalosis.

Gastrointestinal System

1. **Anorexia, nausea, and vomiting:** May occur with acute fluid volume deficit or fluid volume excess.
2. **Thirst:** Symptomatic of increased osmolality or fluid volume deficit.

Laboratory Assessment of Fluid, Electrolyte, and Acid-Base Balance

5

Laboratory tests are vital in the early identification and continuous monitoring of fluid, electrolyte, and acid-base imbalances. Consideration of laboratory results should be included in the nursing assessment of patients at risk for fluid, electrolyte, and acid-base disturbances. The laboratory values that follow are applicable to the adult.

Tests to Evaluate Fluid Status
Serum Osmolality

Normal is 280-300 mOsm/kg.
Serum osmolality measures the solute concentration of the blood. It may be measured directly or estimated by doubling the serum sodium as sodium and its accompanying anions are the primary determinants of serum osmolality. A more exact estimate of serum osmolality considers glucose and urea by using the following formula:

$$\text{Serum osmolality} = 2\,Na^+ + \frac{\text{serum glucose}}{18} + \frac{\text{urea (BUN)}}{2.8}$$

Because glucose and urea are measured by weight (mg/dl), their values must be converted to concentration (number of particles) by dividing their weight per liter of solution by their molecular weight. Hence, glucose is divided by 18 and blood urea nitrogen (BUN) is divided by 2.8.

1. **Factors that may increase serum osmolality:**
   - *Free water loss:* For example, insensible water loss (see Chapter 3, p. 25) for a discussion of insensible water loss).
   - *Diabetes insipidus:* See Chapter 20 for additional information.
   - *Sodium overload:* For example, excessive administration of sodium bicarbonate ($NaHCO_3$).
   - *Hyperglycemia:* See Chapter 20 for more information.

2. **Factors that may decrease serum osmolality:**
   - *Syndrome of inappropriate antidiuretic hormone (SIADH)*: See Chapter 20.
   - *Diuretics.*
   - *Adrenal insufficiency:* See "Addisonian Crisis" in Chapter 20.
   - *Renal failure:* Caused by retention of excess water. See Chapter 22.
   - *Isotonic fluid loss* that is replaced with water or hypotonic fluids: For example, vomiting of isotonic gastric contents with water replacement.

Hematocrit

Normals are 40-54% (males); and 37-47% (females).

Hematocrit measures the volume (percentage) of whole blood that is composed of red blood cells (RBCs). Because hematocrit measures the percentage of cells in relation to plasma, it will be affected by changes in plasma volume. Thus, the hematocrit will increase with dehydration and decrease with overhydration. The hematocrit may remain normal immediately following an acute hemorrhage (the concentration of RBCs to plasma has not changed), but over a period of hours there is a shift of fluid from the interstitial fluid (ISF) to the plasma and the hematocrit drops. The kidneys compensate for the loss of volume by retaining sodium and water.

Urea Nitrogen

Blood Urea Nitrogen (BUN); normal is 6-20 mg/dl.

Urea is produced by the body as a by-product of hepatic protein metabolism. Its primary means of removal from the body is excretion by the kidneys. Urea production occurs at a fairly steady rate so that an increased BUN usually reflects a reduction in renal function. Urea synthesis and excretion can be affected, however, by such additional factors as hydration, protein intake, and tissue catabolism, thereby limiting the usefulness of BUN as an indicator of renal function.

1. **Factors that may increase BUN:**
   - *Decreased renal function:* If the increase in BUN is solely the result of reduced renal function, the serum creatinine level will increase at approximately the same rate (creatinine to BUN ratio will be 1:10-20).
   - *Excessive protein intake.*
   - *GI bleeding:* Owing to digestion of blood in the gut.
   - *Increased tissue catabolism (breakdown):* For example, with fever, sepsis, antianabolic steroid use.
   - *Dehydration:* Urea excretion varies with water excretion. In dehydration, decreased water excretion causes decreased urea excretion.
2. **Factors that may decrease BUN:**
   - *Low protein diet.*
   - *Severe liver disease:* Due to decreased hepatic synthesis.
   - *Volume expansion:* For example, overhydration with IV fluids, pregnancy.

Urine Osmolality

Physiologic range is approximately 50-1400 mOsm/kg; a typical 24-hour specimen is approximately 300-900 mOsm/kg.

This is a measure of the solute concentration of the urine. Unlike plasma, the primary determinants of urinary osmolality are nitrogenous wastes (e.g., urea, creatinine, uric acid). The kidney is capable of excreting a concentrated, yet almost sodium-free, urine. Although the maximum urine osmolality in the adult may be as high as 1400 mOsm/kg, the neonate is capable of concentrating urine to no greater than 500 mOsm/kg and the child to only 700 mOsm/kg.

Note: Urinary values for concentration and composition are normal or abnormal only in relation to what is occurring in the blood. A patient with severe diaphoresis, for example, would be expected to have a relatively high urine osmolality (the kidneys should be compensating for the hypotonic fluid loss by retaining water). In contrast, a patient who has been overhydrated with IV 5 percent dextrose in water (D_5W) would be expected to have a relatively low urine osmolality (the kidneys should be compensating for the excess water intake by excreting a dilute urine). In this case, a relatively high urine osmolality would be abnormal.

1. **Factors that may increase urine osmolality:**
   - *Fluid volume deficit.*
   - *SIADH:* Urine osmolality will be inappropriately high, given the serum osmolality. See Chapter 20 for more information.
2. **Factors that may decrease urine osmolality:**
   - *Fluid volume excess.*
   - *Diabetes insipidus:* See Chapter 20 for additional information.

Urine Specific Gravity

Physiologic range: 1.001-1.040; random specimen with normal fluid intake is approximately 1.010-1.020.

Specific gravity measures the weight of a solution in relation to water (water = 1.000). Urine specific gravity evaluates the kidneys' ability to conserve or excrete water. It is a less reliable indicator of concentration than urine osmolality, because specific gravity is affected both by the weight and number of solutes. The presence in the urine of a few large solutes such as glucose or protein may cause a deceptively high specific gravity. Advantages of the test are that it can be performed quickly, easily, and inexpensively at the bedside by nursing staff. Table 5-1 shows the relationship of osmolality to specific gravity.

Factors that increase and decrease specific gravity are the same as those that affect urine osmolality. Some substances that may give a false high specific gravity include glucose, protein, dextran, radiographic contrast material, and medications such as carbenicillin disodium.

Table 5-1   Relationship of osmolality to specific gravity

Osmolality	Specific Gravity
350 mOsm/kg	≈ 1.010
700 mOsm/kg	≈ 1.020
1050 mOsm/kg	≈ 1.030
1400 mOsm/kg	≈ 1.040 (physiologic maximum for urinary concentration)

Urine Sodium

Random specimen normal ranges from 50-130 mEq/L.

Urine sodium levels vary with sodium intake (e.g., increased intake results in increased excretion) and volume status (e.g., sodium is conserved in the presence of a decreased effective circulating volume). Levels may be measured from 24-hour specimens or from random specimens.

Note: Diuretics and advanced renal failure may increase urine sodium levels.

Clinical applications of urine sodium levels:

- *Evaluation of volume status.*
- *Differential diagnosis of hyponatremia (decreased serum sodium).*
- *Differential diagnosis of acute renal failure.*

Urine sodium, osmolality, and specific gravity may be helpful in differentiating between oliguria caused by decreased effective circulating volume (ECV), and oliguria secondary to acute tubular necrosis (ATN). In volume depletion or decreased ECV, the kidneys are able to respond appropriately by conserving sodium and concentrating urine. Thus urine sodium will be minimal, urine osmolality will exceed plasma osmolality, and urine specific gravity will be greater than 1.015. In ATN (a type of acute renal failure—see Chapter 22) the kidneys lose their ability to conserve sodium and concentrate urine appropriately. The urine osmolality will remain fixed at less than 350 mOsm/kg, the specific gravity will be fixed at approximately 1.010, and urine sodium typically will be greater than 20-40 mEq/L (Table 5-2).

Table 5-2   Urinary values: hypovolemia vs. acute tubular necrosis

Urinary Test	Hypovolemia	Acute Tubular Necrosis
Urine osmolality (mOsm/kg H_2O)	>350	≤350
Urine specific gravity	1.020	Fixed at ≈ 1.010
Urine sodium	<20	>40

Table 5-3   Serum electrolytes: normal values

Na^+	137-147 mEq/L
Cl^-	95-108 mEq/L
K^+	3.5-5.0 mEq/L
HCO_3^-	22-26 mEq/L
Ca^{2+}	8.5-10.5 mg/dl
	4.3-5.3 mEq/L
Mg^{2+}	1.8-3.0 mg/dl
	1.5-2.5 mEq/L
PO_4^{3-}	2.5-4.5 mg/dl
	1.7-2.6 mEq/L

Tests to Evaluate Electrolyte Balance

Refer to Chapters 7-11 for individual discussions of each of the electrolytes. See Table 5-3 for normal values.

Tests to Evaluate Acid-Base Balance
Arterial Blood Gases (ABGs)

ABGs measure the pH, carbon dioxide (CO_2) tension, and oxygen (O_2) tension of arterial blood, and oxygen saturation of hemoglobin. A bicarbonate level of arterial blood also is included in an ABG test and may be measured directly or calculated from pH and carbon dioxide tension of arterial blood ($Paco_2$). ABGs evaluate acid-base balance and pulmonary function. Table 5-4 lists normal ABG values. See Chapter 12 for additional information including a step-by-step guide to ABG analysis.

Table 5-4   Arterial blood gases: normal values

pH	7.35-7.45
$Paco_2$	35-45 mm Hg
Pao_2	80-95 mm Hg
O_2 saturation	95-99%
HCO_3^-	22-26 mEq/L

$Paco_2$ = carbon dioxide tension of arterial blood; Pao_2 = oxygen tension of arterial blood; HCO_3^- = bicarbonate

Carbon Dioxide Content or Total Carbon Dioxide

Normal range is 22-28 mEq/L.
Using a venous blood sample, this test measures carbon dioxide content in all its chemical forms: dissolved CO_2 (Pco_2), bicarbonate (HCO_3^-), and carbonic acid (H_2CO_3). Carbonic acid exists only briefly, and therefore its concentration is negligible. Because dissolved CO_2 accounts for only 1.2 mEq/L, the CO_2 content primarily reflects the bicarbonate level. It will increase in metabolic alkalosis and decrease in metabolic acidosis.

Anion Gap

Normal range is 10 (+ or − 2) mEq/L.
Anion gap reflects the normally unmeasured anions (e.g., phosphates, sulfates, and proteins) in the plasma. Anion gap equals $Na^+ - (Cl^- + HCO_3^-)$. Measurement of the anion gap (Figure 5-1) may be helpful in the differential diagnosis of metabolic acidosis or in identifying hidden metabolic acidosis in certain mixed acid-base disorders.

To understand anion gap, think of the ECF as two equal-sized columns—one containing cations (positively charged ions) and the other containing anions (negatively charged ions). Because electroneutrality is maintained at all times within the body, the number of cations and anions (or the size of the two columns as shown in Figure 5-1) always must be equal. Sodium is the body's primary cation, thus the overall size of Column 1 may be determined by measuring serum sodium. The two primary anions of the ECF are chloride and bicarbonate. Their sum (Cl^- mEq/L

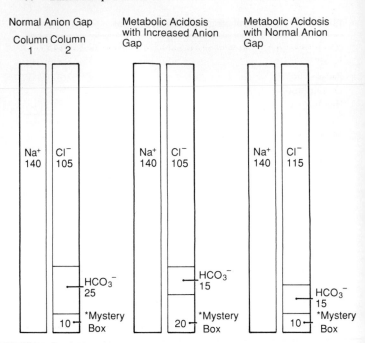

* = Unmeasured Anions ⟶ Anion Gap

Figure 5-1.   Anion gap and metabolic acidosis.

plus HCO_3^- mEq/L) does not completely fill Column 2. The remaining portion of Column 2 (mystery box) represents the normally unmeasured anions of the ECF. This mystery box (anion gap) may be determined by obtaining a serum electrolyte panel and using the following formula:

Anion gap (mystery box) = $Na+ - (Cl^- + HCO_3^-)$.

The size of the anion gap is significant because the causes of metabolic acidosis fall into two categories: (1) those that cause an increase in unmeasured anions and thus increase the mystery box/ anion gap, and (2) those that result from a loss of bicarbonate or an ingestion or administration of acidifying salts and do not alter the mystery box/anion gap. See Tables 5-5 and 5-6, and Chapters 15 and 17 for additional information.

Table 5-5   Causes of metabolic acidosis with a normal anion gap

Loss of HCO_3^-

- Diarrhea
- Lower GI fistulas
- Ureterosigmoidostomy
- Renal tubular acidosis
- Early renal insufficiency
- Diuretics: Acetozolamide (Diamox), triamterene (Dyrenium), spironolactone (Aldactone)

Addition of Acidifying Salts

- Ammonium chloride
- Hyperalimentation fluids without adequate bicarbonate or bicarbonate-producing solutes (e.g., lactate or acetate)
- Lysine hydrochloride
- Arginine hydrochloride

Table 5-6   Causes of metabolic acidosis with an increased anion gap

Retention of Acids

- Renal failure

Ingestion

- Salicylates
- Methanol
- Paraldehyde

Abnormal Production of Acids

- Ketoacidosis
- Lactic acidosis

Urine pH

Random specimen 4.6-8.0.
The kidneys play a critical role in the regulation of acid-base balance by excreting a portion of the hydrogen ions (H^+) produced each day. In spite of a buffering system within the renal tubule,

which allows maximal excretion of H^+ with minimal decrease in urinary pH, the pH of the urine usually is markedly acidic (averaging approximately 6.0). Measurement of urine pH may be useful in determining if the kidneys are responding appropriately to metabolic acid-base imbalances. Urine pH should decrease in metabolic acidosis and increase in metabolic alkalosis. An inappropriately high urine pH in the presence of metabolic acidosis, for example, suggests renal tubular acidosis (a group of disorders that inhibit renal excretion of H^+). An inappropriately low pH in the presence of metabolic alkalosis may signal volume depletion (i.e., sodium bicarbonate is retained as the kidneys attempt to correct the volume deficit by conserving all filtered sodium). Urinary tract infections with pathogens that produce urease cause an alkaline urine due to excess ammonia production. Urine pH should be measured within 1-2 hours of collection. Urine becomes increasingly alkaline as it sits.

Lactic Acid

Normal arterial value is 0.5-1.6 mEq/L; venous is 1.5-2.2 mEq/L.

Lactic acid is a by-product of the anaerobic metabolism of glucose. Normally, the small quantity of lactic acid that is produced daily is immediately buffered by bicarbonate, and lactate is generated. This lactate is then converted to CO_2 and water (H_2O) or glucose by the liver and HCO_3^- is regenerated. Any time there is an excess production of lactic acid (e.g., when there is a decreased oxygen delivery to the tissue) or decreased utilization of lactate, dangerous lactic acidosis may develop.

Factors that may lead to the development of lactic acidosis:

- *Increased production of lactic acid.*
  - Strenuous exercise.
  - Shock.
  - Cardiac arrest.
  - Carbon monoxide poisoning.
  - Hypoxemia.
- *Decreased utilization of lactate.*
  - Liver disease.
  - Severe acidosis.

Related Tests

Creatinine

Normal is 0.6-1.5 mg/dl.
Creatinine is a metabolic waste product produced by the break-down of muscle creatine. The serum creatinine level reflects the balance between production and excretion by the kidneys. Because it is produced at a steady rate dependent on muscle mass and is not affected by diet, hydration, or tissue catabolism, the creatinine level is a more accurate indicator of renal function than BUN. The serum creatinine level will increase as renal function decreases.

Serum Albumin

Normal is 3.5-5.5 g/dl.
Albumin is a small plasma protein produced by the liver that acts osmotically to help hold the intravascular volume in the vascular space. Decreased serum albumin (hypoalbuminemia) may lead to the development of edema due to the movement of water out of the vascular space and into the interstitial space. The edema seen in protein malnutrition occurs due to decreased albumin production.

Factors that may decrease serum albumin:

- *Decreased protein intake:* For example, protein malnutrition.
- *Decreased hepatic synthesis:* For example, cirrhosis.
- *Abnormal urinary loss:* For example, nephrotic syndrome.

DISORDERS OF FLUID, ELECTROLYTE, AND ACID-BASE BALANCE

II

Disorders of Fluid Balance

6

Hypovolemia

Depletion of extracellular fluid (ECF) volume is termed "hypovolemia." It occurs because of abnormal skin, GI, or renal losses; bleeding; decreased intake; or movement of fluid into a nonequilibrating third space (Table 6-1). Depending on the type of fluid lost, hypovolemia may be accompanied by acid-base, osmolar, or electrolyte imbalances. Severe ECF volume depletion can lead to hypovolemic shock. Compensatory mechanisms in hypovolemia include increased sympathetic nervous system stimulation (increased heart rate, inotrophy [cardiac contraction], and vascular resistance), thirst, release of antidiuretic hormone (ADH), and release of aldosterone. Prolonged hypovolemia may lead to the development of acute renal failure (see Chapter 22).

Assessment

1. **Signs and symptoms:** Dizziness, weakness, fatigue, syncope, anorexia, nausea, vomiting, thirst, confusion, constipation, oliguria.
2. **Physical assessment:** Decreased BP, especially when standing (orthostatic hypotension); increased heart rate (HR); poor skin turgor; dry, furrowed tongue; sunken eyeballs; flattened neck veins; increased temperature; and acute weight loss (Table 6-2), except with third spacing. *Infants and children:* Loss of tearing; depressed anterior fontanel.

   The patient in shock will appear pale and diaphoretic with a rapid, thready pulse; supine hypotension; and olig-

Table 6-1   Common disorders associated with third-space* fluid shift

Disorder	Pathophysiologic Process
Peritonitis	Trapping of fluid and electrolytes in the peritoneal cavity owing to damage to or inflammation of the peritoneum. As many as six liters of fluid can accumulate, depending on degree of acuity.
Bowel obstruction	Loss of lower GI fluid due to sequestering of same in the distended bowel. Several liters may accumulate in the intestinal lumen, leading to a dramatic increase in lumen pressure with eventual damage to intestinal mucosa.
Burns	Temporary sequestering of fluid in the interstitial space owing to increased capillary permeability, decreased vascular colloid osmotic pressure.
Ascites	Accumulation of several liters of fluid in the peritoneal cavity, occurring in severe hepatic cirrhosis. Ascites occurs in cirrhosis due to hepatic venous obstruction and retention of sodium and water. Symptomatic hypovolemia is most likely to occur after paracentesis due to rapid reaccumulation of ascitic fluid.
Fractured hip	Loss of intravascular volume due to extensive bleeding into the joint.
Carcinoma	Trapping of fluid in the interstitial space due to lymphatic or venous obstruction.
Major surgery involving extensive tissue trauma	Abnormal sequestration of fluid at the surgical site owing to extensive tissue involvement (e.g., with major abdominal surgery). It also can occur with the loss of ECF into the wall and lumen of the bowel during bowel surgery.

*There is no third space, per se, but rather, it is a concept describing fluid that is temporarily unavailable either to intracellular fluid (ICF) or ECF. Because third-space fluids are unavailable to the body for its use, the patient will exhibit clinical indicators associated with fluid volume deficit, with the exception of weight loss.

Table 6-2   Weight loss as an indicator of ECF deficit in adults and children

Acute Weight Loss	Severity of Deficit
2-5%	Mild
5-10%	Moderate
10-15%	Severe
15-20%	Fatal

Table 6-3   Assessment changes with hypovolemia

Mild Hypovolemia	Moderate Hypovolemia	Severe Hypovolemia
Anorexia	Orthostatic	Supine hypotension
Fatigue	hypotension	Rapid, thready pulse
Weakness	Tachycardia	Cool, clammy skin
	Decreased CVP	Oliguria
	Decreased urine output	Confusion, stupor, coma

uria. See Table 6-3 for assessment changes associated with hypovolemia.

3. **Hemodynamic measurements:** Decreased CVP, decreased pulmonary artery pressure (PAP), decreased cardiac output (CO), decreased mean arterial pressure (MAP), increased systemic vascular resistance (SVR).

4. **History and risk factors:**
   - *Abnormal GI losses:* Vomiting, NG suctioning, diarrhea, intestinal drainage.
   - *Abnormal skin losses:* Excessive diaphoresis secondary to fever or exercise; burns; cystic fibrosis.
   - *Abnormal renal losses:* Diuretic therapy, diabetes insipidus, renal disease (polyuric forms), adrenal insufficiency, osmotic diuresis (e.g., uncontrolled diabetes mellitus, postdye study). See p. 11 for a discussion of osmotic diuresis.
   - *Third spacing or plasma-to-interstitial fluid shift:* Peritonitis, intestinal obstruction, burns, ascites (see Table 6-1).
   - *Hemorrhage.*
   - *Altered intake:* Coma, fluid deprivation.

Diagnostic Tests

1. **Blood urea nitrogen (BUN):** May be elevated due to dehydration, decreased renal perfusion, or decreased renal function.
2. **Hematocrit:** Elevated with dehydration; decreased in the presence of bleeding. Remember that the hematocrit will remain normal immediately following acute hemorrhage but over a period of hours there will be a shift of fluid from the ISF to the plasma and the hematocrit will drop (see Figure 6-1).
3. **Serum electrolytes:** Variable, depending on type of fluid lost. Hypokalemia often occurs with abnormal GI or renal losses. Hyperkalemia occurs with adrenal insufficiency.

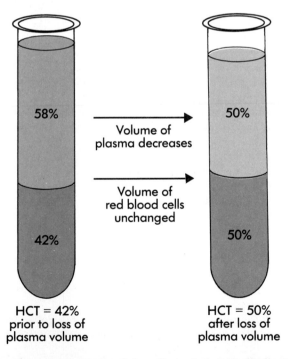

Figure 6-1. An example of the effect of plasma volume loss on hematocrit.

Hypernatremia may be seen with increased insensible or sweat losses and diabetes insipidus. Hyponatremia occurs in most types of hypovolemia due to increased thirst and ADH release, which leads to increased water intake and retention, thus diluting the serum sodium. See discussion of individual electrolyte disorders, Chapters 7 through 11.

4. **Serum total CO_2 (also known as CO_2 content):** Decreased with metabolic acidosis and increased with metabolic alkalosis (see "ABG values," below).

5. **Arterial blood gas (ABG values):** Metabolic acidosis (pH <7.35 and HCO_3^- <22 mEq/L) may occur with lower GI losses, shock, or diabetic ketoacidosis. Metabolic alkalosis (pH >7.45 and HCO_3^- >26 mEq/L) may occur with upper GI losses or diuretic therapy.

6. **Urine specific gravity:** Increased due to the kidneys' attempt to save water; may be fixed at approximately 1.010 in the presence of renal disease; will be decreased in diabetes insipidus.

7. **Urine sodium:** Demonstrates the kidneys' ability to conserve sodium in response to an increased aldosterone level. In the absence of renal disease, osmotic diuresis, or diuretic therapy, it should be <10-20 mEq/L.

8. **Serum osmolality:** Variable, depending on the type of fluid lost and the body's ability to compensate with thirst and ADH.

Collaborative Management

1. **Restoration of normal fluid volume and correction of accompanying acid-base and electrolyte disturbances.** The type of fluid replacement depends on the type of fluid lost and severity of the deficit, serum electrolytes, serum osmolality, and acid-base status.
   - *Dextrose and water:* Provides free water only and will be distributed evenly throughout both ICF and ECF; used to treat total body water deficits only.
   - *Isotonic (normal) saline:* Expands ECF only; does not enter ICF. Usually it is used as an intravascular volume expander or to replace abnormal losses.
   - *Blood and blood components:* Expand only the intravascular portion of ECF.

- *Mixed saline/electrolyte solutions:* Provide additional electrolytes (e.g., potassium and calcium) and a buffer (lactate or acetate). Usually, hypotonic solutions are used as maintenance fluids, whereas isotonic solutions are used as replacement fluids because most abnormal fluid losses are isotonic. See Tables 6-4 and 6-5 and Fluid Therapy section, pp. 80–88, for additional information.

Fluids should be administered rapidly enough and in sufficient quantity to maintain adequate tissue perfusion without overloading the cardiovascular system. The patient's underlying cardiac and renal functions determine how well he or she will tolerate fluid replacement. Thus, the rate of fluid administration should be based both on severity of the loss and the individual's hemodynamic response to volume replacement. During a fluid challenge, volumes of fluid are administered at specific rates and intervals and the patient's hemodynamic response is monitored and documented. Hemodynamic parameters may be prescribed by the physician or, depending on agency policy, determined by a fluid challenge protocol. A typical fluid challenge includes the following steps:

- Baseline vital signs (VS), hemodynamic measurements (e.g., CVP, PAP, and CO) and clinical data (e.g., breath sounds, skin color and temperature, and sensorium) are obtained.
- Initial volume of fluid is administered as prescribed or per protocol (e.g., 100-200 ml NS over 10 minutes).
- Patient is reassessed after 10 minutes.
- If the patient continues to demonstrate signs of hypovolemia (i.e., CVP and PAP remain low), additional fluid may be administered per MD or agency protocol.
- If the CVP or PAP increases too rapidly (e.g., >2 mm Hg for the CVP or >3 mm Hg for the PAP), fluid administration is discontinued and the patient is reassessed after 10 minutes. If after 10 minutes the CVP or PAP has dropped and the patient shows no signs of fluid overload, fluid administration is resumed.

- Fluid administration is continued until the desired hemo-
    dynamic parameters are achieved or a specific volume
    has been infused (e.g., 500-1000 ml). The fluid chal-
    lenge should be discontinued if the patient shows signs
    of fluid volume excess (e.g., crackles [rales], increased
    HR, increased respiratory rate [RR]) or there is a rapid
    increase in CVP or PAP.

    Note: Continued nursing assessment is essential during
    and after the fluid challenge.

2. **Restoration of tissue perfusion in hypovolemic shock.**
    The potential for the development of shock is dependent
    on both the volume lost (usually greater than 25% of the
    intravascular volume) and the rapidity of the loss. In turn,
    successful treatment depends on rapid volume replace-
    ment. Initially, hemorrhagic shock is treated with an iso-
    tonic electrolyte solution, and packed RBCs are given as
    the hematocrit drops. A balanced electrolyte solution
    (e.g., Ringer's lactate) is recommended because 0.9%
    NaCl contains excessive amounts of sodium and chloride
    (see Table 6-4). Fresh frozen plasma is used to replace
    clotting factors when clotting disorders are present or mas-
    sive transfusions are necessary. Human albumin, dextran,
    or hetastarch also may be used to supplement volume re-
    placement (see Table 6-5). Their use, however, remains
    controversial. Autotransfusion has become an increasingly
    common therapy in hemorrhagic shock. Autologous blood
    drained from a sterile body cavity is retransfused within 4
    hours of collection *via* an autotransfusion device.

3. **Oral rehydration in pediatric diarrhea:** See discussion at
    end of chapter, p. 88.

4. **Treatment of underlying cause.**

Text continued on p. 66.

Table 6-4 Composition and use of commonly prescribed crystalloid solutions

Solution	Glucose g/L	Electrolyte Composition mEq/L					Tonicity/mOsm/L	Indications and Considerations*
		Na$^+$	K$^+$	Ca^{2+}	Cl$^-$	HCO$_3$$^-$		
Dextrose in water								
1. 5%	50	—	—	—	—	—	Isotonic/278	▪ Provides free water necessary for renal excretion of solutes ▪ Used to replace water losses and treat hypernatremia ▪ Provides 170 kcal/L ▪ Does not provide any electrolytes
2. 10%	100	—	—	—	—	—	Hypertonic/556	▪ Provides free water only, no electrolytes ▪ Provides 340 kcal/L
Saline								
3. 0.45%	—	77	—	—	77	—	Hypotonic/154	▪ Provides free water in addition to Na$^+$ and Cl$^-$ ▪ Used to replace hypotonic fluid losses

4. 0.9%	—	154	154	—	—	Isotonic/308	■ Used as a maintenance solution although it does not replace daily losses of other electrolytes ■ Provides no calories ■ Used to expand intravascular volume and replace ECF losses ■ Only solution that may be administered with blood products ■ Contains Na^+ and Cl^- in excess of plasma levels ■ Does not provide free water, calories, or other electrolytes ■ May cause intravascular overload or hyperchloremic acidosis
5. 3.0%	—	513	513	—	—	Hypertonic/1026	■ Used to treat symptomatic hyponatremia

Table continued on p. 60.

Table 6-4 (*continued*)

Solution	Glucose g/L	Electrolyte Composition mEq/L					Tonicity/mOsm/L	Indications and Considerations*
		Na$^+$	K$^+$	Ca^{2+}	Cl$^-$	HCO$_3^-$		
								■ Must be administered slowly and with extreme caution because it may cause dangerous intravascular volume overload and pulmonary edema
Dextrose in saline								
6. 5% in 2.225%	50	38.5	—	—	38.5	—	Isotonic/355	■ Provides Na$^+$, Cl$^-$, and free water ■ Used to replace hypotonic losses and treat hypernatremia ■ Provides 170 kcal/L
7. 5% in 0.45%	50	77	—	—	77	—	Hypertonic/432	■ Same as 0.45% NaCl except that it provides 170 kcal/L
8. 5% in 0.9%	50	154	—	—	154	—	Hypertonic/586	■ Same as 0.9% NaCl except that it provides 170 kcal/L

Multiple electrolyte solutions

9. Ringer's	—	147	4	5	156	—	Isotonic/309

- Similar in composition to plasma except that it has excess Cl^-, no Mg^{2+}, and no HCO_3^-
- Does not provide free water or calories
- Used to expand the intravascular volume and replace ECF losses

10. Lactated Ringer's (Hartmann's solution)	—	130	4	3	109	28†	Isotonic/274

- Similar in composition to normal plasma except that it does not contain Mg^{2+}
- Used to treat losses from burns and lower GI tract
- May be used to treat mild metabolic acidosis but should not be used to treat lactic acidosis
- Does not provide free water or calories

*Modified from Rose DB, Clinical pathology of acid-base and electrolyte disorders, ed 3, New York, 1989, McGraw-Hill, Inc.
†In the form of lactate.

Table 6-5 Composition and use of commonly prescribed colloid solutions

Solution	Composition	Volume	Indications and Considerations
Blood and blood components			
Whole blood	RBCs, WBCs, platelets, plasma, and some clotting factors	Approximately 500 ml/unit	▪ Used to treat acute massive blood loss, although rarely required as most hemorrhagic episodes may be treated with packed RBCs and crystalloids ▪ In the stable patient should increase hematocrit 3% or hemaglobin 1 g/dl/unit ▪ Requires ABO and Rh compatibility ▪ Administer with 0.9% NaCl only
Packed RBCs	RBCs and some plasma ($\approx$ 20%), platelets, and WBCs	250-350 ml/unit	▪ Indicated in patients requiring increased O_2 carrying capacity, but not necessarily volume expansion ▪ Less plasma proteins and clotting factors than whole blood ▪ Requires ABO and Rh compatibility

			▪ Specially prepared leukocyte depleted units may be used to decrease the risk of febrile, nonhemolytic transfusion reactions
Fresh frozen plasma	Plasma, plasma proteins, and clotting factors	200 ml	▪ Used to restore clotting factors in situations of known deficiency ▪ Although helpful in restoring volume, it should not be used solely for volume expansion ▪ Should be used promptly after thawing to prevent deterioration of clotting factors ▪ Requires ABO compatibility
Plasma protein fraction	5% solution of human plasma proteins (85% albumin, 15% globulins)	250–500 ml units 290 mOsm/L	▪ Used to expand plasma volume ▪ Greater risk of hypersensitivity reactions than with pure albumin solutions ▪ Does not require typing ▪ Virtually no risk of hepatitis or HIV infection

Table continued on p. 64.

Table 6-5 (continued)

Solution	Composition	Volume	Indications and Considerations
Albumin	Human albumin in a buffered saline solution; available in 5% or 25% concentrations	5% = 250 and 300 ml units 300 mOsm/L 25% = 50 and 100 ml units 1500 mOsm/L	■ Used to expand plasma volume and increase plasma oncotic pressure ■ 25% albumin will expand the vascular volume 3–4 ml for each ml administered ■ Does not require typing ■ Virtually no risk of hepatitis or HIV infection ■ 25% should be used with caution in persons with cardiac or renal failure due to the risk of intravascular fluid (IVF) overload

Plasma substitutes

Dextran 70	6% solution of polysaccharide (average molecular weight of 70,000) combined with saline or dextrose and water	500 ml/unit

- Used for rapid volume expansion
- Less expensive than blood products
- May cause bleeding tendencies, interference with crossmatching, and release of histamine

Hetastarch	6% solution of hydroxyethyl starch in saline	500 ml/unit 310 mOsm/L

- Used for rapid volume expansion
- Less expensive than blood products
- May cause bleeding tendencies and circulatory overload
- Should be used with caution in persons with renal failure due to decreased urinary excretion of hetastarch

Nursing Diagnoses and Interventions

Fluid volume deficit related to abnormal loss of body fluids or reduced intake

Desired outcomes: Patient attains adequate intake of fluid and electrolytes as evidenced by urine output ≥30 ml/hr, stable weight, specific gravity 1.010-1.030, no clinical evidence of hypovolemia (furrowed tongue, etc.), BP within patient's normal range, CVP 2-6 mm Hg, and HR 60-100 bpm. Serum sodium is 137-147 mEq/L and hematocrit and BUN are within patient's normal range. For patients in critical care the following are attained: PAP 20-30/8-15 mm Hg and CO 4-7 L/min.

1. Monitor I&O hourly. Initially, intake should exceed output during therapy. Alert physician to urine output 30 ml/hr or less for two consecutive hours. Measure urine specific gravity every 8 hours. Expect it to decrease with therapy.

2. Monitor VS and hemodynamic pressures for signs of continued hypovolemia. Be alert to decreased BP and CVP and increased HR and SVR. For critical patients, also be alert to decreased PAP, CO, and MAP and to increased SVR.

3. Weigh patient daily. Daily weights are the single most important indicator of fluid status because acute weight changes are indicative of fluid changes. For example, a 2 kg loss of weight equals a 2 L fluid loss. Weigh patient at the same time of day (preferably before breakfast) on a balanced scale, with patient wearing approximately the same clothing. Document type of scale used (i.e., standing, bed, chair).

4. Administer oral and IV fluids as prescribed. Document response to fluid therapy. Monitor for signs and symptoms of fluid overload or too rapid fluid administration: crackles, shortness of breath (SOB), tachypnea, tachycardia, increased CVP, increased PAP, neck vein distention, and edema. If the patient is symptomatic of any of the above signs and symptoms, follow agency protocol for fluid challenge.

5. Monitor patient for hidden fluid losses. For example, measure and document abdominal girth or limb size, if indicated.

6. Notify physician of decreases in hematocrit that may signal bleeding. Remember that hematocrit will decrease in the dehydrated patient as he or she becomes rehydrated. Decreases in hematocrit associated with rehydration may be accompanied by decreases in serum sodium and BUN.

7. Place shock patient in a supine position with the legs elevated at 45 degrees to increase venous return. This position returns approximately 500 ml of blood pooled in the veins of the legs to the central circulation. Avoid the Trendelenburg position because this causes abdominal viscera to press on the diaphragm, thereby impairing ventilation. If shock occurs secondary to hemorrhage, draw blood for possible type and crossmatch and ensure that the patient has a No. 16-18 gauge IV access to allow rapid administration of packed red blood cells. Insert a Foley catheter to monitor hourly urine output, because hourly output reflects the adequacy of fluid replacement.

8. Securely tape all nonLuer–Lok connections on IV lines to prevent bleeding caused by accidental disconnection. Luer-Lok-type connections *must* be used on arterial lines because of the high risk of hemorrhage and on central lines because of the additional risk of air embolus.

Altered cerebral, renal, and peripheral tissue perfusion related to hypovolemia.

Desired outcome: Patient has adequate perfusion as evidenced by alertness, warm and dry skin, BP within patient's normal range, HR <100 beats per minute (bpm), urinary output ≥ 30 ml/hr for 2 consecutive hours, capillary refill <2 seconds, and peripheral pulses $>2^+$ on a $0-4^+$ scale.

1. Monitor for signs of decreased cerebral perfusion: vertigo, syncope, confusion, restlessness, anxiety, agitation, excitability, weakness, nausea, and cool and clammy skin. Alert physician to worsening symptoms. Document response to fluid therapy.

2. Protect patients who are confused, dizzy, or weak. Keep side rails up and bed in lowest position with wheels locked. Assist with ambulation in step-down units. Raise patient to sitting or standing positions slowly. Monitor for indicators of orthostatic hypotension: decreased BP, in-

creased heart rate, dizziness, and diaphoresis. If symptoms occur, return patient to supine position.

3. To avoid unnecessary vasodilatation, treat fevers promptly.
4. Reassure patient and significant others that sensorium changes will improve with therapy.
5. Monitor I&O and alert physician to urine output <30 ml/hr for 2 consecutive hours. Prolonged reduction in renal perfusion may result in ischemic damage to the kidneys and acute renal failure.
6. Evaluate capillary refill, noting whether it is brisk (<2 seconds) or delayed (≥2 seconds). Notify physician if refill is delayed.
7. Palpate peripheral pulses bilaterally in arms and legs (radial, brachial, dorsalis pedis, and posterior tibial). Use a Doppler if unable to palpate pulses. Rate pulses on a 0-4+ scale. Notify physician if pulses are absent or barely palpable. **Note:** Abnormal pulses also may be caused by a local vascular disorder.

For additional nursing diagnoses, see specific medical disorder, electrolyte imbalance, or acid-base disturbance.

Patient-Family Teaching Guidelines

Give patient and significant others verbal and written instructions for the following:

1. Signs and symptoms of hypovolemia.
2. Importance of maintaining adequate intake, especially in small children and the elderly, who are more likely to develop dehydration.
3. Medications: name, purpose, dosage, frequency, precautions, and potential side effects.

Hypervolemia

Expansion of ECF volume is termed "hypervolemia." It occurs whenever there is (1) chronic stimulus to the kidney to save sodium and water; (2) abnormal renal function, with reduced excretion of sodium and water; (3) excessive administration of IV fluids; or (4) interstitial-to-plasma fluid shift. Hypervolemia can lead to heart failure and pulmonary edema (see Chapter 21), especially in the patient with cardiovascular dysfunction. Compensatory mechanisms for hypervolemia include the release of atrial natriuretic peptide (ANP—see Chapter 2), leading to increased filtration and excretion of sodium and water by the kidneys and decreased release of aldosterone and ADH. Abnormalities in electrolyte homeostasis, acid-base balance, and osmolality often accompany hypervolemia.

Assessment

1. **Signs and symptoms:** SOB, orthopnea.
2. **Physical assessment:** Edema, weight gain, increased BP (decreased BP as the heart fails), bounding pulses, ascites, crackles (rales), rhonchi, wheezes, distended neck veins, moist skin, tachycardia, gallop rhythm.
3. **Hemodynamic measurements:** Increased CVP, PAP, and MAP.
4. **History and risk factors**
   - *Retention of sodium and water:* Heart failure, cirrhosis, nephrotic syndrome, excessive administration of glucocorticosteroids.
   - *Abnormal renal function:* Acute or chronic renal failure with oliguria.
   - *Excessive administration of IV fluids.*
   - *Interstitial-to-plasma fluid shift:* Remobilization of fluid after treatment of burns, excessive administration of hypertonic solutions (e.g., mannitol, hypertonic saline) or colloid oncotic solutions (e.g., albumin).

Diagnostic Tests

Laboratory findings are variable and usually nonspecific.

1. **Hematocrit:** Decreased due to hemodilution.
2. **BUN:** Increased in renal failure.
3. **Arterial blood gas (ABG) values:** May reveal hypoxemia (decreased Pao_2) and alkalosis (increased pH and decreased $Paco_2$) in the presence of pulmonary edema.
4. **Serum sodium and serum osmolality:** Will be decreased if hypervolemia occurs as a result of excessive retention of water (e.g., in chronic renal failure.)
5. **Urinary sodium:** Elevated if the kidney is attempting to

Table 6-6   Foods that are high in sodium content

Bouillon	Olives
Celery	Pickles
Cheeses	Preserved meat
Dried fruits	Salad dressings and prepared
Frozen, canned, or packaged	sauces
foods	Sauerkraut
Monosodium glutamate	Snack foods (e.g., crackers,
(MSG)	chips, pretzels)
Mustard	Soy sauce

excrete excess sodium. Urinary sodium will not be elevated in conditions with secondary hyperaldosteronism (e.g., congestive heart failure, cirrhosis, nephrotic syndrome) because hypervolemia occurs secondary to a chronic stimulus to the release of aldosterone.

6. **Urine specific gravity:** Decreased if the kidney is attempting to excrete excess volume. May be fixed at 1.010 in acute renal failure.

7. **Chest x-ray:** May reveal signs of pulmonary vascular congestion.

Collaborative Management

The goal of therapy is to treat the precipitating problem and return ECF to normal. Treatment may include the following:

1. **Restriction of sodium and water:** See Table 6-6 for a list of foods high in sodium.

2. **Diuretics.**

3. **Dialysis or continuous arteriovenous hemofiltration:** In renal failure or life-threatening fluid overload.

Note: Also see specific discussions of "Acute Renal Failure," p. 218, and "Burns," p. 233.

 ## Nursing Diagnoses and Interventions

Fluid volume excess related to excessive fluid or sodium intake or compromised regulatory mechanism

Desired outcomes: Patient is normovolemic as evidenced by adequate urinary output of at least 30-60 ml/hr, specific gravity of

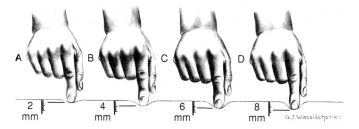

Figure 6-2.   Assessment of pitting edema: **A**, +1; **B**, +2; **C**, +3; **D**, +4. (From Bobak IM and Jensen MD: Essentials of maternity nursing, ed 3, St. Louis, 1990, Mosby−Year Book.)

approximately 1.010-1.020, stable weights, and absence of edema. BP is within patient's normal range, CVP is 2-6 mm Hg, and HR is 60-100 bpm. In addition, for critical care patients PAP is 20-30/8-15 mm Hg, MAP is 70-105 mm Hg, and CO is 4-7 L/min.

1. Monitor I&O hourly. With the exception of oliguric renal failure, urine output should be >30-60 ml/hr. Measure urine specific gravity every shift. If patient is diuresing, specific gravity should be <1.010-1.020.

2. Observe for and document presence of edema: pretibial, sacral, periorbital. Rate pitting on a 1-4 scale (Figure 6-2).

3. Weigh patient daily. Daily weights are the single most important indicator of fluid status. For example, a 2 kg acute weight gain is indicative of a 2 L fluid gain. Weigh patient at the same time each day (preferably before breakfast) on a balanced scale, with patient wearing approximately the same clothing. Document type of scale used (i.e., standing, bed, chair).

4. Obtain an accurate dietary history, and limit sodium intake as prescribed by physician (see Table 6-6). Consider use of salt substitutes. **Note:** Salt substitutes contain potassium and may be contraindicated in patients with renal failure or in patients receiving potassium-sparing diuretics (e.g., spironolactone, triamterene). Incorporate cultural considerations when providing dietary counseling.

5. Limit fluids as prescribed. Offer a portion of allotted fluids

as ice chips to minimize patient's thirst. Teach patient and significant others the importance of fluid restriction and how to measure fluid volume.
6. Provide oral hygiene at frequent intervals to keep oral mucous membrane moist and intact.
7. Document response to diuretic therapy. Many diuretics (e.g., furosemide, thiazides) cause hypokalemia. Observe for indicators of hypokalemia: muscle weakness, dysrhythmias (especially premature ventricular contractions [PVCs] and ECG changes—flattened T wave, presence of U waves). See "Hypokalemia," p. 98. Potassium-sparing diuretics (e.g., spironolactone, triamterene) may cause hyperkalemia: weakness, ECG changes (e.g., peaked T wave, prolonged PR interval, widened QRS). See "Hyperkalemia," p . 103. Notify physician of significant findings.
8. Observe for physical indicators of overcorrection and dangerous volume depletion secondary to therapy: vertigo, weakness, syncope, thirst, confusion, poor skin turgor, flat neck veins, acute weight loss. Monitor VS and hemodynamic parameters for signs of volume depletion occurring with therapy: decreased BP, CVP, PAP, MAP, and CO; increased HR. Alert physician to significant changes or findings.

Impaired gas exchange related to alveolar-capillary membrane changes secondary to pulmonary vascular congestion occurring with ECF expansion
Desired outcomes: Patient has adequate gas exchange as evidenced by RR ≤20 breaths/min, HR ≤100 bpm, and Pao_2≥80 mm Hg. Patient does not exhibit crackles, gallops, or other clinical indicators of pulmonary edema. For patients in critical care, PAP is ≤30/15 mm Hg.
1. Acute pulmonary edema is a potentially life-threatening complication of hypervolemia. Monitor patient for indicators of pulmonary edema including air hunger, anxiety, cough with production of frothy sputum, crackles (rales), rhonchi, tachypnea, tachycardia, gallop rhythm, and elevation of PAP and pulmonary artery wedge pressure (PAWP).
2. Monitor ABGs for evidence of hypoxemia (decreased Pao_2) and respiratory alkalosis (increased pH and de-

creased Paco$_2$). Increased oxygen requirements are indicative of increasing pulmonary vascular congestion.
3. Keep patient in semi-Fowler's or position of comfort to minimize dyspnea. Avoid restrictive clothing.
4. Administer O$_2$ according to unit protocol or physician's prescription.

High risk for impaired skin and tissue integrity related to edema secondary to fluid volume excess
Desired outcome: Patient's skin remains free of erythema, sores, and ulcerations.
1. Assess and document circulation to extremities at least every shift. Note color, temperature, capillary refill, and peripheral pulses. Determine whether capillary refill is brisk (<2 seconds) or delayed (≥2 seconds). Palpate peripheral pulses bilaterally in the arms and legs (radial, brachial, dorsalis pedis, and posterior tibial). Use Dopper if unable to palpate pulses. Notify physician if capillary refill is delayed or pulses are absent.
2. Turn and reposition patient at least every 2 hours to minimize tissue pressure.
3. Check tissue areas at risk with each position change (e.g., heels, sacrum, and other areas over bony prominences).
4. Use special air or fluidized mattress to minimize pressure.
5. Support arms and hands on pillows and elevate legs to decrease dependent edema (unless pulmonary edema or heart failure is present).
6. Treat decubitus ulcers with occlusive dressings (e.g., Duoderm, Op-Site, Tegaderm) as per unit protocol. Notify physician of the presence of sores, ulcers, or areas of tissue breakdown in patients who are at increased risk for infection (e.g., diabetics, immunosuppressed individuals, those with renal failure).

Patient-Family Teaching Guidelines

Give patient and significant others verbal and written instructions for the following:
1. Signs and symptoms of hypervolemia.
2. Symptoms that necessitate physician notification after hospital discharge: SOB, chest pain, new pulse irregularity.

3. Low sodium diet, if prescribed; use of salt substitute; and avoiding foods that are high in sodium. (See Table 6-6.)
4. Medications, including name, purpose, dosage, frequency, precautions, and potential side effects; signs and symptoms of hypokalemia if patient is taking diuretics.
5. Importance of fluid restriction if hypervolemia continues.
6. Importance of daily weights.

Edema Formation

Edema occurs as a result of expansion of the interstitial fluid volume and is defined as a palpable swelling of the interstitial space that is either localized (e.g., thrombophlebitis with venous obstruction) or generalized (e.g., cardiac failure). Severe generalized edema is termed *anasarca*. Edema may develop any time there is an alteration in capillary hemodynamics favoring either increased formation or decreased removal of interstitial fluid (Figure 6-3). Increased capillary hydrostatic pressure from vol-

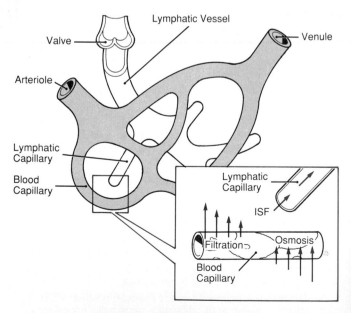

Figure 6-3.   Capillary diagram.

ume expansion or venous obstruction, or increased capillary permeability owing to burns, allergy, or infection, causes an increase in interstitial fluid volume. Decreased removal of interstitial fluid occurs when there is an obstruction to lymphatic outflow or a decrease in plasma oncotic pressure (remember that the plasma proteins help to hold the vascular volume in the vascular space). Furthermore, retention of sodium and water by the kidneys enhances and maintains generalized edema. This may be due to a decreased ability to excrete sodium and water (overflow) as in renal failure, or an increased stimulus to conserve sodium and water (underfilling). In heart failure, for example, impaired cardiac function leads to a reduction in CO with a drop in ECV, which in turn stimulates the kidneys to conserve sodium and water *via* the reninangiotensin system. As the patient with heart failure retains volume, the venous circuit expands, capillary hydrostatic pressure increases, and edema is formed. The edema seen in nephrotic syndrome and hepatic cirrhosis (ascites, [see Chapter 24]) is the result of both underfilling and overflow.

Assessment

Generalized edema usually is most evident in dependent areas. The ambulatory patient will exhibit pretibial or ankle edema, whereas the patient restricted to bed will exhibit sacral edema. Generalized edema also may present around the eyes (periorbital) or in the scrotal sac due to the low tissue pressures in these areas. Sacral edema may be identified by pressing the index finger firmly into the sacral tissue and maintaining the pressure for several seconds. If a pit remains after the finger has been withdrawn, edema is present. Pitting also may be assessed over the tibia or ankle. Rate pitting according to severity (Figure 6-2). See Chapter 21 for a discussion of pulmonary edema.

Collaborative Management

1. **Treatment of the primary problem:** For example, digitalis for patients with congestive heart failure.
2. **Mobilization of edema:** For example, with bed rest and supportive hose.
3. **Dietary restrictions of sodium and fluids:** In addition, hidden sodium sources (e.g., medications) should be avoided.

4. **Diuretic therapy:** See below.
5. **Dialysis or continuous arteriovenous hemofiltration:** In renal failure or life-threatening fluid overload.
6. **Abdominal paracentesis:** For the treatment of severe ascites that adversely affects cardiopulmonary functioning.

Diuretic Therapy

Diuretics reduce edema by inhibiting the reabsorption of sodium and water by the kidneys. Diuretics also may induce the loss of other important electrolytes and alter acid-base balance. Although retention of sodium and water by the kidneys is an important component in the development of edema, not all edematous states require treatment with diuretics. Reduction in ECV and alterations in electrolyte balance caused by diuretics may be detrimental. Patients with hepatic cirrhosis, for example, may develop hepatic coma or hepatorenal syndrome with overuse of diuretics owing to diuretic-induced hypokalemia, metabolic alkalosis, and rapid fluid removal. The majority of edematous patients, however, may benefit by the judicious use of diuretics.

The quantity and characteristics of the diuresis varies, depending on the type of diuretic and its site of action within the renal tubule (Figure 6-4 and Table 6-7). Although there are some complications of diuretic therapy that are common to all or most diuretics (see discussion below), the specifics of nursing care will depend on the type of diuretic the patient is receiving (Table 6-7).

Complications of Diuretic Therapy

1. **Volume abnormalities:** Volume depletion owing to over-diuresis. Monitor patients for signs of fluid volume deficit: dizziness, weakness, fatigue, postural hypotension.
2. **Electrolyte disturbances:**
   - *Hypokalemia:* Occurs due to increased secretion and excretion of potassium by the kidneys. It may occur with all the diuretics except for those that work in the late distal tubule. Hypokalemia can be avoided by giving a potassium-sparing diuretic (see Table 6-7) or a potassium supplement. Monitor patients for indicators of hy-

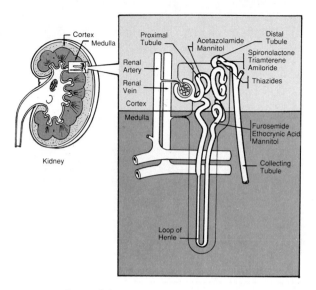

Figure 6-4.   Sites of diuretic action.

pokalemia (e.g., fatigue, muscle weakness, leg cramps, and irregular pulse).

- *Hyperkalemia:* Occurs owing to decreased secretion and excretion of potassium by the kidneys. It may occur with diuretics that work in the late distal tubule (see Table 6-7). The potassium-sparing diuretics should not be given to patients with decreased renal function (because of the increased risk of hyperkalemia) or in patients receiving a potassium supplement. Monitor patient for indicators of hyperkalemia: irritability, anxiety, abdominal cramping, muscle weakness (especially in the lower extremities), and ECG changes (see Chapter 8 for additional information).

- *Hyponatremia:* Occurs because of an increased stimulus to the release of ADH secondary to a reduction in effective circulating volume (remember that ADH affects the reabsorption and retention of water only). Monitor patient for indicators of hyponatremia: irritability, apprehension, and dizziness.

Table 6-7   Diuretic action

Diuretic (by Site of Action)	Potency	Characteristic of Diuresis
Proximal tubule		
Acetazolamide (Diamox)*	Weak	$NaHCO_3$ diuresis with the loss of additional Na^+, Cl^-, and K^+
Proximal tubule and loop		
Mannitol†	Moderate	Osmotic diuresis with the loss of water in excess of Na^+ and Cl^-
Loop of Henle		
Furosemide (Lasix)‡	Strong	Large diuresis (may affect 25-30% of filtered load of sodium) with loss of Na^+, Cl^-, and K^+
Ethacrynic acid (Edecrin)¶	Strong	Same as above
Early distal tubule		
Thiazides (Diuril, Hydrodiuril, Esidrix)#	Moderate	Diuresis affecting up to 5% of filtered load of sodium, with loss of Cl^- and K^+
Metolazone (Zaroxolyn)#	Similar to thiazides	
Chlorthalidone (Hygrotin)#	Similar to thiazides	

Late distal tubule— Potassium-sparing diuretics

Spironolactone (Aldactone)**	Weak	Blocks the action of aldosterone, with loss of Na^+ and Cl^- but not K^+
Triamterene (Dyrenium)**	Weak	Weak diuresis with loss of Na^+ and Cl^- but not K^+. Does not depend on the presence of aldosterone.

Clinical indications and nursing considerations:

*May be used in the treatment of metabolic alkalosis or in combination with other diuretics to treat refractory edema. It is most commonly used to treat glaucoma because it decreases the formation of aqueous humor. It is contraindicated in patients with acidosis. Monitor patients for hypokalemia (see Chapter 8).

†May cause hyperosmolality and circulatory overload owing to the osmotic shift of fluid out of the cells and into the interstitium and intravascular space. Use with caution in patients with decreased cardiac function. Monitor for signs of circulatory overload (e.g., crackles, SOB, tachycardia). It may be used in the treatment of early acute renal failure.

‡Used to treat edema of CHF and advanced renal failure. It may be used alone or in combination with mannitol or dopamine to reverse early acute renal failure. It is effective in the treatment of acute pulmonary edema owing to its diuretic and direct venous vasodilatory actions. Do not give IV faster than 4-5 mg/min because of the risk of deafness. Stop the infusion and notify the physician if the patient complains of ringing in the ears. Monitor for hypokalemia (see Chapter 8) and volume depletion (see this chapter).

¶Same as ‡.

#Often used to treat hypertension owing to diuretic action and antihypertensive effect, which is unrelated to diuretic action. This group of diuretics has the most nondiuresis-related side effects (e.g., decreased release of insulin, hyperlipidemia, skin rashes). Monitor patient for hypokalemia (see Chapter 8), hyperglycemia, and volume depletion (see this chapter). These diuretics also may cause hyperuricemia and hypercalcemia (see Chapter 9).

**May be combined with the thiazide diuretics for increased diuretic action and less hypokalemia. These diuretics may cause hyperkalemia (see Chapter 8).

- *Hypomagnesemia:* Occurs owing to decreased reabsorption and increased excretion of magnesium by the kidneys. This may occur with the loop and thiazide type diuretics and will contribute to the development of hypokalemia. Monitor patients for indicators of hypomagnesemia: confusion, cramps, and dysrhythmias.

3. **Acid-base disturbances:**
   - *Metabolic alkalosis:* May be caused by the loop and thiazide type diuretics due to an increased secretion and excretion of hydrogen by the kidneys and the contraction of the ECF around the existing bicarbonate (contraction alkalosis). Monitor patients for indicators of metabolic alkalosis: muscular weakness, dysrhythmias, apathy, and confusion.
   - *Metabolic acidosis:* May occur owing to increased loss of bicarbonate in the urine with acetazolamide. Monitor patients for indicators of metabolic acidosis: tachypnea, fatigue, confusion. Metabolic acidosis also may occur with the potassium-sparing diuretics.

4. **Other metabolic complications:**
   - *Azotemia:* This is increased retention of metabolic wastes (e.g., urea and creatinine) owing to a reduction in effective circulating volume with decreased perfusion of the kidneys and decreased excretion of metabolic wastes. Alert physician to changes in BUN and serum creatinine levels.
   - *Hyperuricemia:* Occurs due to increased reabsorption and decreased excretion of uric acid by the kidneys. Alert physician to patient complaints of gouty type pain. This condition usually is problematic only in patients with preexisting gout.

Fluid Therapy

The goals of IV fluid are to maintain or restore normal fluid volume and electrolyte balance and to provide a means of administering medications quickly and efficiently. An additional concern is that of nutrition. Unfortunately, routine IV fluids (i.e., 5% dextrose solutions) contain only enough carbohydrates to minimize tissue breakdown and starvation. They do not provide ade-

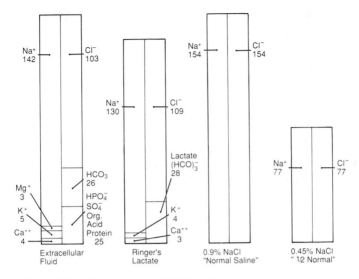

Figure 6-5.   Comparison of ECF and three common IV solutions (mEq/L).

quate calories and essential amino acids needed for tissue synthesis. Five percent dextrose solutions, for example, supply only 170 calories per liter, whereas the average patient on bed rest requires a minimum of 1500 calories per day. Patients should not be maintained solely on 5% dextrose solutions for longer than a few days. See Chapter 26 for a discussion of nutritional therapies and total parenteral nutrition (TPN).

The type of IV fluid prescribed for volume replacement or maintenance depends on several factors, including the type of fluid lost and the patient's nutritional needs, serum electrolytes, serum osmolality, and acid-base balance. See Figure 6-5 for a comparison of lactated Ringer's solution, 0.9% NaCl, and 0.45 NaCl to ECF fluid.

Text continued on p. 86.

Table 6-8   Acute transfusion reactions

Reaction	Cause	Clinical Manifestations	Management	Prevention
Acute hemolytic	Infusion of ABO-incompatible whole blood, RBCs, or components containing 10 ml or more of RBCs. Antibodies in the recipient's plasma attach to antigens on transfused RBCs causing RBC destruction.	Chills, fever, low back pain, flushing, tachycardia, tachypnea, hypotension, vascular collapse, hemoglobinuria, hemoglobinemia, bleeding, acute renal failure, shock, cardiac arrest, death.	Treat shock, if present. Draw blood samples for serologic testing slowly to avoid hemolysis from the procedure. Send urine specimen to the laboratory. Maintain BP with IV colloid solutions. Give diuretics as prescribed to maintain urine flow. Insert indwelling catheter or measure voided amounts to monitor hourly urine output. Dialy-	Meticulously verify and document patient identification from sample collection to component infusion.

			sis may be required if renal failure occurs. Do not transfuse additional RBC-containing components until transfusion service has provided newly crossmatched units.
Febrile, nonhemolytic (most common)	Sensitization to donor white blood cells, platelets, or plasma proteins.	Sudden chills and fever (rise in temperature of greater than 1° C), headache, flushing, anxiety, muscle pain.	Give antipyretics as prescribed—avoid aspirin in thrombocytopenic patients. **Do not restart transfusion.** Consider leukocyte-poor blood products (filtered, washed, or frozen).
Mild allergic	Sensitivity to foreign plasma proteins.	Flushing, itching, urticaria (hives).	Give antihistamine as directed. If symptoms are mild and transient, transfusion may be restarted slowly. Treat prophylactically with antihistamines.

Table continued on p. 84.

Table 6-8 (continued)

Reaction	Cause	Clinical Manifestations	Management	Prevention
			Do not restart transfusion if fever or pulmonary symptoms develop.	
Anaphylactic	Infusion of IgA proteins to IgA-deficient recipient who has developed IgA antibody.	Anxiety, urticaria, wheezing, progressing to cyanosis, shock, and possible cardiac arrest.	Initiate CPR, if indicated. Have epinephrine ready for injection (0.4 ml of a 1:1,000 solution subcutaneously or 0.1 ml of 1:1,000 solution diluted to 10 ml with saline for IV use). **Do not restart transfusion.**	Transfuse extensively washed RBC products, from which all plasma has been removed. Alternatively, use blood from IgA deficient donor.

Circulatory overload	Fluid administered faster than the circulation can accommodate.	Cough, dyspnea, pulmonary congestion (rales), headache, hypertension, tachycardia, distended neck veins.	Place patient upright with feet in dependent position. Administer prescribed diuretics, oxygen, morphine. Phlebotomy may be indicated.	Adjust transfusion volume and flow rate based on patient size and clinical status. Have transfusion service divide unit into smaller aliquots for better spacing of fluid input.
Sepsis	Transfusion of contaminated blood components.	Rapid onset of chills, high fever, vomiting, diarrhea, and marked hypotension and shock.	Obtain culture of patient's blood and send bag with remaining blood to transfusion service for further study. Treat septicemia as directed—antibiotics, IV fluids, vasopressors, steroids.	Collect, process, store, and transfuse blood products according to blood banking standards and infuse within 4 hrs of starting time.

From National Blood Resource Education Programs, Transfusion therapy guidelines for nurses, September, 1990, NIH Publication No. 90-2668a.

Commonly Prescribed Intravenous Fluids

IV fluids are divided into two major categories: crystalloids and colloids. *Crystalloid solutions* contain only electrolytes and glucose, substances that are not restricted to the intravascular space. Therefore, these solutions will expand the entire extracellular space. Depending on their sodium content, crystalloids also may expand the intracellular fluid (ICF) volume. Isotonic NaCl (0.9%) will expand only the ECF, whereas hypotonic NaCl solutions and dextrose and water solutions expand all fluid compartments. Table 6-4 compares commonly prescribed crystalloid solutions.

Colloids are solutions that contain cells, proteins, or synthetic macromolecules that do not readily cross the capillary membrane. These solutions remain within the vascular space and, depending on their concentration, may cause an osmotic shift of fluids from the interstitum into the intravascular space. Table 6-5 compares commonly prescribed colloid solutions. Blood is the most commonly administered colloid. See Table 6-8, p. 82, for common causes of blood transfusion reactions and the box below for nursing management of transfusion reactions.

When a Transfusion Reaction Occurs

1. STOP THE TRANSFUSION.
2. Keep the IV open with 0.9% normal saline.
3. Report the reaction to both the transfusion service and attending physician immediately.
4. Do clerical check at bedside of identifying tags and numbers.
5. Treat symptoms per physician's order and monitor vital signs.
6. Send blood bag with attached administration set and labels to the transfusion service.
7. Collect blood and urine samples and send to laboratory.*
8. Document thoroughly on transfusion reaction form and in patient chart.

---

*Check with the transfusion service to determine the specific blood and urine samples needed to evaluate reactions.

From National Blood Resource Education Programs, Transfusion therapy guidelines for nurses, September, 1990, NIH Publication No. 90-2668a.

Table 6-9 Composition of oral rehydration solutions

Formula	Na$^+$ (mEq/L)	K$^+$ (mEq/L)	Cl$^-$ (mEq/L)	Base (mEq/L)	Carbohydrate (g/L)
Lytren (Mead-Johnson)	50	25	45	30 (citrate)	20 (dextrose, corn syrup, solids)
Pedialyte	45	20	35	30 (citrate)	25 (dextrose)
Rehydrolyte	75	20	65	30 (citrate)	25 (dextrose)
Infalyte powder (Pennwalt)	50	20	40	30 (bicarbonate)	20 (glucose)
WHO (World Health Organization)	90	20	80	30 (bicarbonate)	18 (dextrose)

From Whaley L. and Wong D: Nursing care of infants and children, ed 4, St Louis, 1991, Mosby–Year Book.

Oral Rehydration in Pediatric Diarrhea

Oral rehydration solutions have been developed to treat fluid deficit associated with diarrhea, a common source of abnormal fluid loss in infancy and early childhood. These solutions contain varying amounts of glucose, sodium, and potassium and some form of buffer. The glucose concentration of oral rehydration solutions is significant because of the relationship of glucose and sodium reabsorption in the gut. Maximal sodium and water absorption is believed to occur with glucose concentrations of 10-25 g/L. Commonly available fluids, such as cola drinks, ginger ale, and apple juice, often are prescribed to replace fluids lost in mild episodes of diarrhea. However, these are poor choices for fluid replacement in prolonged or severe diarrhea because of their high-glucose and low-electrolyte concentrations. See Table 6-9 for examples of oral rehydration solutions.

Disorders of Sodium Balance

7

Sodium plays a vital role in maintaining concentration and volume of extracellular fluid (ECF). It is the main cation of ECF and the major determinant of ECF osmolality. Under normal conditions, ECF osmolality can be estimated by doubling the serum sodium value. Sodium imbalances usually are associated with parallel changes in osmolality. Sodium also is important in maintaining irritability and conduction of nerve and muscle tissue and assists with the regulation of acid-base balance.

The average daily intake of sodium far exceeds the body's normal daily requirements. The kidneys are responsible for excreting the excess and are capable of conserving sodium avidly during periods of extreme sodium restriction. Sodium concentration is maintained *via* regulation of water intake and excretion. If serum sodium concentration is decreased (hyponatremia), the kidneys respond by excreting water. Conversely, if serum sodium concentration is increased (hypernatremia), serum osmolality increases, stimulating the thirst center and causing an increased release of antidiuretic hormone (ADH) by the posterior pituitary gland. ADH acts on the kidneys to conserve water. The adrenal cortical hormone, aldosterone, is an important regulator of sodium and ECF volume. The release of aldosterone causes the kidney to conserve sodium and water, thereby increasing ECF volume. Because changes in serum sodium levels typically reflect changes in water balance, gains or losses of total body sodium are not necessarily reflected by the serum sodium level. Normal serum sodium is 137-147 mEq/L.

Hyponatremia

Hyponatremia (serum sodium <137 mEq/L) can occur because of a net gain of water or loss of sodium-rich fluids that are replaced by water. Clinical indicators and treatment depend on the cause of hyponatremia and whether or not is is associated with a normal, decreased, or increased ECF volume. For more information, see "Syndrome of Inappropriate Antidiuretic Hormone (SIADH)," p. 212, "Congestive Heart Failure," p. 215, "Acute Renal Failure," p. 218, and "Burns," p. 233.

 Assessment

1. **Signs and symptoms:**
   Note: Neurologic symptoms usually do not occur until the serum sodium level has dropped to approximately 120-125 mEq/L.
   - *Hyponatremia with decreased ECF volume:* Irritability, apprehension, dizziness, personality changes, postural hypotension, dry mucous membranes, cold and clammy skin, tremors, seizures, coma.
   - *Hyponatremia with normal or increased ECF volume:* Headache, lassitude, apathy, confusion, weakness, edema, weight gain, elevated BP, muscle cramps, convulsions, coma.

2. **Hemodynamic measurements:**
   - *Decreased ECF volume:* Evidence of hypovolemia including decreased central venous pressure (CVP), pulmonary artery pressure (PAP), cardiac output (CO), mean arterial pressure (MAP), increased systemic vascular resistance (SVR).
   - *Increased ECF volume:* Evidence of hypervolemia including increased CVP, PAP, MAP.

3. **History and risk factors:**
   - *Decreased ECF volume:*
     —GI losses: Diarrhea, vomiting, fistulas, (NG) suction.
     —Renal losses: Diuretics, salt-wasting kidney disease, adrenal insufficiency.
     —Skin losses: Burns, wound drainage.
   - *Normal/increased ECF volume:*
     —Syndrome of inappropriate antidiuretic hormone: Excessive production of antidiuretic hormone (see Chapter 20).

—Edematous states: Congestive heart failure, cirrhosis, nephrotic syndrome.

—Excessive administration of hypotonic IV fluids.

—Oliguric renal failure.

—Primary psychogenic polydipsia.

Note: Hyperlipidemia, hyperproteinemia, and hyperglycemia may cause a pseudohyponatremia. Hyperlipidemia and hyperproteinemia reduce the total percentage of plasma that is water. The sodium/water ratio of the plasma does not change, but the plasma sodium level is reduced because there is a reduction in plasma water. With hyperglycemia, the osmotic action of the elevated glucose causes a shift of water out of the cells and into the ECF, thus diluting the existing sodium. For every 100 mg/dl glucose is elevated, sodium is diluted by 1.6 mEq/L.

Diagnostic Tests

1. **Serum sodium:** Will be <137 mEq/L.
2. **Serum osmolality:** Decreased, except in cases of pseudo-hyponatremia, azotemia, or ingestion of toxins that increase osmolality (e.g., ethanol, methanol).
3. **Urine specific gravity:** Decreased because of the kidneys' attempt to excrete excess water. In SIADH, the urine will be inappropriately concentrated.
4. **Urine sodium:** Decreased (usually <20 mEq/L) except in SIADH and adrenal insufficiency.

Collaborative Management

The goal of therapy is to get the patient out of immediate danger (i.e., return sodium to >120 mEq/L) and then gradually return sodium to a normal level and restore normal ECF volume.

Hyponatremia with Reduced Extracellular Fluid Volume

1. **Replacement of sodium and fluid losses.**
2. **Replacement of other electrolyte losses** (e.g., potassium, bicarbonate).

3. **IV hypertonic saline:** If serum sodium is dangerously low or the patient is very symptomatic.

Hyponatremia with Expanded Extracellular Fluid Volume

1. **Removal or treatment of underlying cause.**
2. **Furosemide** (thiazide diuretics should be avoided).
3. **Water restriction.**
4. **Hemofiltration.**

Nursing Diagnoses and Interventions

Fluid volume deficit related to abnormal fluid loss; **Fluid volume excess** related to excessive intake of hypotonic solutions or increased retention of water

Desired outcomes: Patient is normovolemic as evidenced by heart rate (HR) 60-100 bpm, respiratory rate (RR) 12-20 breaths/min, BP within patient's normal range, and CVP 2-6 mm Hg. For critical care patients, PAP is 20-30/8-15 mm Hg.

1. If patient is receiving hypertonic saline, assess carefully for signs of intravascular fluid overload: tachypnea, tachycardia, shortness of breath (SOB), crackles, rhonchi, increased CVP, increased PAP, gallop rhythm, and increased BP. If given too rapidly, hypertonic saline may cause crenation (shriveling) of the red blood cells in addition to causing an osmotic shift of fluid into the vascular space.
2. For other interventions, see "Hypovolemia, p. 66 for **Fluid volume deficit**; see "Hypervolemia," p. 70 for **Fluid volume excess.**

Sensory-perceptual alterations secondary to a serum sodium level <120-125 mEq/L

Desired outcome: Patient verbalizes orientation to person, place, and time.

1. Assess and document level of consciousness (LOC), orientation, and neurologic status with each vital sign (VS) check. Reorient patient as necessary. Alert MD to significant changes.
2. Inform patient and significant others that altered sensorium is temporary and will improve with treatment.

3. Keep side rails up and bed in lowest position, with wheels locked.
4. Use reality therapy such as clocks, calendars, and familiar objects; keep these items at the bedside within patient's visual field.
5. If seizures are expected, pad side rails and keep an airway at the bedside.

Patient-Family Teaching Guidelines

Give patient and significant others verbal and written instructions for the following:

1. Medications, including drug name, purpose, dosage, frequency, precautions, and potential side effects. Teach signs and symptoms of hypokalemia if patient is taking diuretics and provide examples of foods that are high in potassium (see Table 8-1).
2. Fluid restriction, if prescribed. Teach patient that a portion of fluid allotment can be taken as ice or Popsicles to minimize thirst.
3. Signs and symptoms of hypovolemia if hypernatremia is related to abnormal fluid losses.

Hypernatremia

Hypernatremia (serum sodium level >147 mEq/L) may occur with water loss, water deprivation, or sodium gain. Because sodium is the major determinant of ECF osmolality, hypernatremia always causes hypertonicity. In turn, hypertonicity causes a shift of water out of the cells, which leads to cellular dehydration.

Assessment

1. **Signs and symptoms:** Intense thirst, fatigue, restlessness, agitation, coma. Symptomatic hypernatremia occurs only in individuals who do not have access to water or who have an altered thirst mechanism (e.g., infants, the elderly, those who are comatose).
2. **Physical assessment:** Low-grade fever, flushed skin, peripheral and pulmonary edema (sodium gain); postural hy-

potension (water loss); increased muscle tone and deep tendon reflexes.

3. **Hemodynamic measurements:** Variable
   - *Sodium excess:* Increased CVP and PAP.
   - *Water loss:* Decreased CVP and PAP. The volume effects of water loss are minimized due to movement of water out of the cells secondary to hypernatremia-induced hypertonicity.

4. **History and risk factors:**
   - *Sodium gain:* IV administration of hypertonic saline or sodium bicarbonate, increased oral intake, primary aldosteronism, saltwater near-drowning, drugs such as sodium polystyrene sulfonate (Kayexalate).
   - *Water loss:* Increased insensible and sensible fluid loss (e.g., diaphoresis, respiratory infection), diabetes insipidus (see Chapter 20), or osmotic diuresis (e.g., hyperglycemia).

Diagnostic Tests

1. **Serum sodium:** Will be >147 mEq/L.
2. **Serum osmolality:** Increased due to elevated serum sodium.
3. **Urine specific gravity and osmolality:** Increased because of the kidneys' attempt to retain water; will be decreased in diabetes insipidus.
4. **Dehydration test:** Water is withheld for 16-18 hours. Serum and urine osmolality are then checked 1 hour after administration of ADH. This test is used to identify the etiology of polyuric syndromes (e.g., central versus nephrogenic diabetes insipidus).

Collaborative Management

1. **IV or oral water replacement:** To treat water loss. If sodium is >160 mEq/L, IV D_5W or hypotonic saline is given to replace pure water deficit.
2. **Diuretics in combination with oral or IV water replacement:** To treat sodium gain.

Note: Hypernatremia is corrected slowly, over approximately 2 days, to avoid too great a shift of water into brain cells, which could cause cerebral edema.

3. **Desmopressin acetate (DDAVP):** To treat central diabetes insipidus.
4. **Removal of cause** (e.g., medications such as lithium) in nephrogenic diabetes insipidus.

Nursing Diagnoses and Interventions

High risk for injury related to altered sensorium secondary to primary hypernatremia or cerebral edema occurring with too rapid correction of hypernatremia
Desired outcomes: Patient does not exhibit evidence of injury due to altered sensorium or seizures. Patient can verbalize orientation to person, place, and time.

1. Cerebral edema may occur if hypernatremia is corrected too rapidly. Monitor serial serum sodium levels; notify MD of rapid decreases.
2. Assess patient for indicators of cerebral edema: lethargy, headache, nausea, vomiting, increased BP, widening pulse pressure, decreased pulse rate, and seizures.
3. Assess and document LOC, orientation, and neurologic status with each VS check. Reorient patient as necessary. Alert MD to significant changes.
4. Inform patient and significant others that altered sensorium is temporary and will improve with treatment.
5. Keep side rails up and bed in lowest position, with wheels locked.
6. Use reality therapy, such as clocks, calendars, and familiar objects; keep these items at the bedside within patient's visual field.
7. If seizures are anticipated, pad side rails and keep an airway at the bedside.

See "Hypovolemia," p. 66 for **Fluid volume deficit** (applicable to hypernatremia caused by water loss); see "Hypervolemia," p. 70 for **Fluid volume excess** (applicable to hypernatremia caused by sodium gain).

Patient-Family Teaching Guidelines

Give patient and significant others verbal and written instructions for the following:

1. Medications, including drug name purpose, dosage, frequency, precautions, and potential side effects. Teach

signs and symptoms of hypokalemia if patient is taking diuretics and review foods that are high in potassium (see Table 8-1).
2. Signs and symptoms of hypovolemia, if hypernatremia is related to abnormal fluid loss.

Disorders of Potassium Balance

8

Potassium is the primary intracellular cation, and it plays a vital role in cell metabolism. A relatively small amount (approximately 2%) of potassium is located within the extracellular fluid (ECF) and is maintained within a narrow range. The vast majority of the body's potassium is located within the cells. Because the ratio of ICF to ECF potassium helps determine the resting membrane potential of nerve and muscle cells, an alteration in the plasma potassium level may adversely affect neuromuscular and cardiac function.

Distribution of potassium between ECF and intracellular fluid (ICF) is affected by ECF pH, as well as by several hormones, including insulin, epinephrine, and aldosterone. Increases in these hormones cause an increased movement of potassium into the cells. Acute changes in serum pH are accompanied by reciprocal changes in serum potassium concentration. In acidosis, for example, excess hydrogen ions move into the cells to be buffered. To maintain electrical neutrality within the cell, another positive ion (e.g., potassium) must move out. In alkalosis the reverse occurs. Hydrogen ions shift out of the cell and potassium ions shift in to replace them.

The body gains potassium through foods (primarily meats, fruits, and vegetables) and medications. In addition, ECF gains potassium any time there is a breakdown of cells (tissue catabolism) or movement of potassium out of the cells. However, an elevated serum potassium level usually does not occur unless there is a concomitant reduction in renal function. Potassium is lost from the body through the kidneys, GI tract, and skin. Potassium may be lost from ECF because of an intracellular shift or tissue anabolism.

The kidneys are the primary regulators of potassium balance. They do this by adjusting the amount of potassium that is excreted in the urine. As the serum potassium level rises after a potassium load, so does the level in the renal tubular cell. This creates a concentration gradient favoring the movement of potassium into the renal tubule with the loss of potassium in the urine. The presence of aldosterone also increases the excretion of potassium. Thus, conditions that increase aldosterone levels (e.g., administration of corticosteroids or postsurgical stress) may increase urinary excretion of potassium. The kidneys are unable to conserve potassium as avidly as sodium and a significant amount of potassium still may be lost in the urine in the presence of potassium depletion. Normal serum potassium is 3.5-5.0 mEq/L.

Hypokalemia

Hypokalemia occurs because of a loss of potassium from the body or a movement of potassium into the cells and is rarely due to inadequate intake alone. **Note:** Changes in serum potassium levels reflect changes in ECF potassium, not necessarily changes in total body levels.

 ## Assessment

1. **Signs and symptoms:** Fatigue, muscle weakness, leg cramps, soft and flabby muscles, nausea, vomiting, ileus, paresthesias, enhanced digitalis effect, decreased urine concentration (e.g., with polyuria).
2. **Physical assessment:** Decreased bowel sounds owing to smooth muscle weakness, weak and irregular pulse, decreased reflexes, and decreased muscle tone.
3. **History and risk factors:**
   - *Reduction in total body potassium:*
     —Hyperaldosteronism (e.g., congenital adrenal hyperplasia).
     —Diuretics or abnormal urinary losses.
     —Increased GI losses, especially gastric losses (e.g., pyloric stenosis).
     —Increased loss through diaphoresis.

Note: Poor dietary intake may contribute to, but rarely will cause, hypokalemia. Hypokalemia may develop in the patient who is maintained on parenteral fluids with inadequate replacement of potassium.

- *Intracellular shift:*
  - Increased insulin (e.g., from total parenteral nutrition).
  - Alkalosis or after correction of acidosis (e.g., treatment of diabetic ketoacidosis [DKA]).
  - During periods of tissue repair after burns, trauma, or starvation. Usually, this is accompanied by inadequate intake or replacement of potassium.

Diagnostic Tests

1. **Serum potassium:** Values will be <3.5 mEq/L.
2. **Arterial blood gases (ABGs):** May show metabolic alkalosis (increased pH and HCO_3^-) because hypokalemia usually is associated with this condition.
3. **Electrocardiogram (ECG):** ST-segment depression, flattened T wave, presence of U wave, ventricular dysrhythmias (Figure 8-1). **Note:** Hypokalemia potentiates the effects of digitalis. ECG may reveal signs of digitalis toxicity in spite of a normal serum digitalis level.

Collaborative Management

1. **Treatment of underlying cause.**
2. **Replacement of potassium:** Either by mouth (PO) (*via* increased dietary intake or medication) or IV. The usual dose is 40-80 mEq/day in divided doses. IV potassium is necessary if hypokalemia is severe or the patient is unable to take potassium orally. IV potassium should not be administered at rates >10-20 mEq/hr or in concentrations >30-40 mEq/L unless hypokalemia is severe, because this can result in life-threatening hyperkalemia. If potassium is administered *via* a peripheral line, the rate of administration may need to be reduced to prevent irritation of vessels. Patients receiving 10-20 mEq/hr should be on a continuous cardiac monitor. The development of peaked T waves suggests the presence of hyperkalemia and requires immediate MD notification. Potassium never may be given as an IV push.

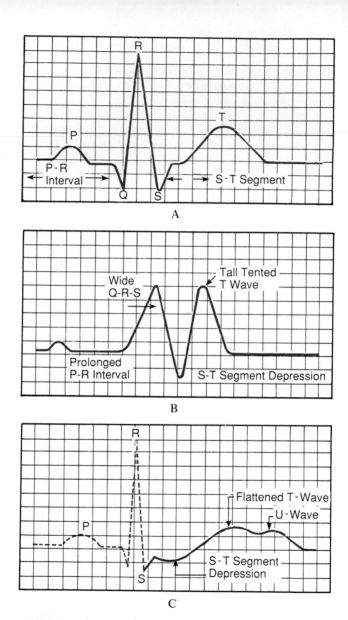

Figure 8-1. **A,** Normal electrocardiographic tracing; **B,** Serum potassium level above normal; **C,** Serum potassium level below normal.

3. **Potassium-sparing diuretics:** May be given in place of oral potassium supplements.
4. **Potassium chloride salt substitute:** May be used to supplement potassium intake (one teaspoon equals approximately 60 mEq potassium chloride).

Nursing Diagnoses and Interventions

Decreased cardiac output related to electrical factors (risk of ventricular dysrhythmias) secondary to hypokalemia or too rapid correction of hypokalemia with resulting hyperkalemia
Desired outcomes: ECG shows normal configuration and absence of ventricular dysrhythmias. Pulse rate and rhythm are normal for the patient. Serum potassium levels are within normal range (3.5-5.0 mEq/L).

1. Administer IV potassium supplement as prescribed. Avoid giving IV potassium chloride at a rate faster than recommended, as this can lead to life-threatening hyperkalemia (see Collaborative Management). Do not add potassium chloride to IV solution containers in the hanging position because this can cause layering of the medication. Instead, invert the solution container before adding the medication and mix well. **Note:** IV potassium chloride can cause local irritation of veins and chemical phlebitis. Assess IV insertion site for erythema, heat, or pain. Alert MD to symptoms. Irritation may be relieved by applying an ice bag, giving mild sedation, or numbing insertion site with small amount of local anesthetic. Phlebitis may necessitate changing of IV site.
2. Administer oral potassium supplements as prescribed. **Note:** Oral supplements may cause GI irritation. Administer with a full glass of water or fruit juice; encourage patient to sip slowly. Alert MD to symptoms of abdominal pain, distention, nausea, or vomiting. Do not switch potassium supplements without MD prescription.
3. Encourage intake of foods high in potassium (see Table 8-1). Salt substitutes may be used as an inexpensive potassium supplement.
4. Monitor Intake and output (I&O)-hourly. Alert MD to urine output <30 ml/hr. Unless severe, symptomatic hypokalemia is present, potassium supplements should not be

Table 8-1 Foods high in potassium

Apricots	Nuts
Artichokes	Oranges, orange juice
Avocado	Potatoes
Banana	Prune juice
Cantaloupe	Pumpkin
Carrots	Rhubarb
Chocolate	Spinach
Dried beans, peas	Swiss chard
Dried fruit	Sweet potatoes
Mushrooms	Tomatoes, tomato juice, tomato sauce
	Turnips

given if the patient has an inadequate urine output because hyperkalemia can develop rapidly in patients with oliguria (<15-20 ml/hr). Alert MD to elevated blood urea nitrogen (BUN) or creatinine levels.

5. Monitor for the presence of an irregular pulse or pulse deficit (a discrepancy between the apical and radial pulse rates). Alert MD to changes.

6. Physical indicators of abnormal potassium levels are difficult to identify in the patient who is critically ill. Monitor ECG for signs of continuing hypokalemia (ST-segment depression, flattened T wave, presence of U wave, ventricular dysrhythmias) or hyperkalemia (tall, thin T waves; prolonged PR interval; ST depression; widened QRS; loss of P wave), which may develop during potassium replacement. (See Figure 8-1.)

7. Monitor serum potassium levels carefully, especially in individuals at risk for developing hypokalemia, such as patients taking diuretics or receiving NG suction.

8. Administer potassium cautiously in patients receiving potassium-sparing diuretics (e.g., spironolactone or triamterene) because of the potential for the development of hyperkalemia.

9. Because hypokalemia can potentiate the effects of digitalis, monitor patients receiving digitalis for signs of increased digitalis effect: multifocal or bigeminal PVCs, par-

oxysmal atrial tachycardia with varying AV block, Wenckebach (type I AV) heart block.

Ineffective breathing pattern related to weakness or paralysis of respiratory muscles secondary to *severe* hypokalemia (potassium <2-2.5 mEq/L)
Desired outcome. Patient has effective breathing pattern as evidenced by normal respiratory depth, pattern, and rate of 12-20 breaths/min.

1. If patient is exhibiting signs of worsening hypokalemia, be aware that severe hypokalemia can lead to weakness of respiratory muscles, resulting in shallow respirations and eventually, apnea and respiratory arrest. Assess character, rate, and depth of respirations. Alert MD promptly if respirations become rapid and shallow.
2. Keep manual resuscitator at patient's bedside if severe hypokalemia is suspected.
3. Reposition patient every 2 hours to prevent stasis of secretions; suction airway as needed.

Patient-Family Teaching Guidelines

Give patient and significant others verbal and written instructions for the following:

1. Medications, including name, purpose, dosage, frequency, precautions, and potential side effects. Teach patient the importance of taking prescribed potassium supplements if taking diuretics or digitalis. Review the indicators of digitalis toxicity.
2. Indicators of hypokalemia and hyperkalemia.
3. Foods that are high in potassium (see Table 8-1); use of salt substitute to supplement potassium, if appropriate.

Hyperkalemia

Hyperkalemia (serum potassium level >5.0 mEq/L) occurs because of an increased intake of potassium, a decreased urinary excretion of potassium, or movement of potassium out of the cells. **Note:** Changes in serum potassium levels reflect changes in ECF potassium, not necessarily changes in total body levels. In diabetic ketoacidosis, for example, a large quantity of potassium may be lost in the urine owing to the glucose-induced osmotic diuresis. Although there may be a significant reduction in total body potassium levels, the patient initially may present with a normal or elevated potassium. This occurs because of the shift of potassium out of the cells secondary to acidosis, lack of insulin, and increased tissue catabolism. For additional information, see Chapter 20.

Assessment

1. **Signs and symptoms:** Irritability, anxiety, abdominal cramping, diarrhea, weakness (especially of lower extremities), paresthesias.
2. **Physical assessment:** Irregular pulse; cardiac standstill may occur at levels >8.5 mEq/L.
3. **History and risk factors:**
   - *Inappropriately high intake of potassium:* Usually, IV potassium delivery.
   - *Decreased excretion of potassium:* For example, with renal disease, use of potassium-sparing diuretics, or adrenal insufficiency (Addison's disease).
   - *Movement of potassium out of the cells:* For example, with acidosis, insulin deficiency, tissue catabolism (e.g., occurring with fever, sepsis, trauma, surgery, or hemolysis).

Diagnostic Tests

1. **Serum potassium:** Will be >5.0 mEq/L. **Note:** Several factors may cause a falsely high serum potassium owing to increased release of intracellular potassium in the laboratory specimen (e.g., a high platelet count, prolonged use of a tourniquet at the time of venipuncture, hemolysis of the blood specimen, or delayed separation of plasma and cells).
2. **ABGs:** May show metabolic acidosis (decreased pH and bicarbonate ion [HCO_3^-]) since hyperkalemia often occurs with acidosis.
3. **Diagnostic ECG:** Progressive changes include tall, thin T

waves; prolonged PR interval; ST depression; widened QRS; loss of P wave. Eventually, QRS becomes widened further and cardiac arrest occurs (see Figure 8-1)

Collaborative Management

The goal is to treat the underlying cause and return the serum potassium level to normal.

Subacute

1. **Cation exchange resins (e.g., Kayexalate):** Given either orally, nasogastrically, or *via* retention enema to exchange sodium for potassium in the bowel. The solution is usually combined with sorbitol to prevent constipation from the Kayexalate and induce diarrhea, thus increasing potassium loss in the bowels. **Note:** Kayexalate may bind with other cations in the GI tract and contribute to the development of hypomagnesemia or hypocalcemia.
2. **Reduced potassium intake:** A diet avoiding high potassium content foods (See Table 8-1). Special intravenous or enteral formulas may be designed for patients with renal failure.

Acute

1. **IV calcium gluconate:** To counteract the neuromuscular and cardiac effects of hyperkalemia. Serum potassium levels will remain elevated. Calcium chloride also may be used. **Note:** Calcium chloride and calcium gluconate are *not* interchangeable. Although both come in 10 ml ampules, calcium gluconate contains only 4.5 mEq of calcium, whereas calcium chloride contains 13.6 mEq of calcium.
2. **IV glucose and insulin:** To shift potassium into the cells. This reduces serum potassium temporarily (approximately 6 hours). Usually hypertonic glucose (either an amp of $D_{50}W$ or 250-500 ml of $D_{10}W$) is given with regular insulin.
3. **Sodium bicarbonate:** To shift potassium into the cells. Reduces serum potassium temporarily (for approximately 1-2 hours). **Note:** The effects of calcium, glucose and insulin,

and sodium bicarbonate are temporary. Usually, it is necessary to follow these medications with a therapy that removes potassium from the body, for example, dialysis or administration of cation exchange resins.

4. **Dialysis:** To remove potassium from the body. Dialysis is the most effective means of removing excess potassium.

ndx: Nursing Diagnoses and Interventions

Decreased cardiac output related to electrical factors (risk of ventricular dysrhythmias) secondary to severe hyperkalemia or too rapid correction of hyperkalemia with resulting hypokalemia
Desired outcomes: ECG shows no evidence of ventricular dysrhythmias related to hypokalemia (U wave, PVCs) or hyperkalemia (peaked T wave). Serum potassium levels are within normal range (3.5-5.0 mEq/L).

1. Monitor I&O. Alert MD to urine output <30 ml/hr. Oliguria increases the risk for developing hyperkalemia.
2. Monitor for indicators for hyperkalemia (e.g., irritability, anxiety, abdominal cramping, diarrhea, weakness of lower extremities, paresthesias, irregular pulse). Also be alert to indicators of hypokalemia (e.g., fatigue, muscle weakness, leg cramps, nausea, vomiting, decreased bowel sounds, paresthesias, weak and irregular pulse) following treatment. Assess for hidden sources of potassium: medications (e.g. potassium penicillin G); banked blood (the older the blood, the greater the amount of potassium owing to the release of potassium as RBCs die and break down); salt substitute; GI bleeding; or conditions causing increased catabolism, such as infection or trauma.
3. Monitor serum potassium levels, especially in patients at risk of developing hyperkalemia, such as individuals with renal failure. Notify MD of levels above or below normal range.
4. Physical indicators of abnormal potassium levels are difficult to identify in the patient who is critically ill. Monitor ECG for signs of hypokalemia (ST-segment depression, flattened T waves, presence of U wave, ventricular dysrhythmias), which may develop secondary to therapy, or continuing hyperkalemia (tall, thin T waves; prolonged PR interval; ST depression; widened QRS; loss of P wave).

Notify MD *stat* if ECG changes occur. ECG changes at a given potassium level will be less dramatic in the chronic renal patient who develops hyperkalemia more slowly. See Figure 8-1 for ECG changes with hypo- and hyperkalemia.

5. Administer calcium gluconate as prescribed, giving it cautiously in patients receiving digitalis because digitalis toxicity can occur. **Note:** Do not add calcium gluconate to solutions containing sodium bicarbonate because precipitates may form. However, IV glucose and sodium bicarbonate ($NaHCO_3$) may be combined without harmful precipitate. Insulin should be given separately. For more information about calcium administration, see "Hypocalcemia," p. 110.

6. If administering cation exchange resins by enema, encourage patient to retain the solution for at least 30-60 minutes to ensure therapeutic effects.

Patient-Family Teaching Guidelines

Give patient and significant others verbal and written instructions for the following:

1. Medications, including name, purpose, dosage, frequency, precautions, and potential side effects.

2. Indicators of both hypokalemia and hyperkalemia. Alert patient to the following signs and symptoms that necessitate immediate medical attention: weakness, pulse irregularities, and fever or other indicator of infection. Teach patient and significant others how to measure pulse rate and detect irregularities.

3. Foods high in potassium, which should be avoided (see Table 8-1). Remind patient that salt substitute and "Lite" salt also should be avoided. Fruits that are relatively low in potassium include apples, grapes, and cranberries.

4. Importance of preventing recurrent hyperkalemia; review potential causes.

Disorders of Calcium Balance

9

Calcium, one of the body's most abundant ions, primarily is combined with phosphorus to form the mineral salts of the bones and teeth. In addition, calcium exerts a sedative effect on nerve cells and has important intracellular functions, including development of the cardiac action potential and contraction of muscles. Less than 1% of the body's calcium is contained within extracellular fluid (ECF), yet this concentration is regulated carefully by parathyroid hormone and calcitonin. Parathyroid hormone is released by the parathyroid gland in response to a low serum calcium level. It increases resorption of bone (movement of calcium and phosphorus out of the bone); activates vitamin D, which increases the absorption of calcium from the GI tract; and stimulates the kidneys to conserve calcium and excrete phosphorus. Calcitonin is produced by the thyroid gland when serum calcium levels are elevated. It inhibits bone resorption.

The ECF gains calcium from intestinal absorption of dietary calcium and resorption of bones. It is lost from the ECF *via* secretion into the GI tract, urinary excretion, and deposition in the bone; and a small amount is lost in sweat.

Calcium is present in three different forms in the plasma: ionized, bound, and complexed. Approximately half of the plasma calcium is free, ionized calcium. Slightly less than half the plasma calcium is bound to protein, primarily to albumin. The remaining small percentage is combined with nonprotein anions, such as phosphate, citrate, and carbonate. Only the ionized calcium is physiologically important. The percentage of calcium that is ionized is affected by plasma pH, phosphorus, and albumin levels. Therefore, these factors must be considered when evaluating total calcium levels.

The relationship between ionized calcium and plasma pH is reciprocal: an increase in pH decreases the percentage of calcium that is ionized. Patients with alkalosis (an increased pH), for example, may show signs of hypocalcemia despite a normal total calcium level (bound, complexed, and ionized). The relationship between plasma phosphorus and ionized calcium is also reciprocal. Changes in plasma albumin level will affect total serum calcium level without changing the level of free calcium. In hypoalbuminemia less protein is available to bind with calcium, and the total calcium level drops; however, the level of ionized calcium is unchanged.

Hypocalcemia

Symptomatic hypocalcemia may occur because of a reduction of total body calcium or a reduction of the percentage of calcium that is ionized. Total calcium levels may be decreased due to increased calcium loss, reduced intake secondary to altered intestinal absorption, or altered regulation (e.g., hypoparathyroidism). Elevated phosphorus levels and decreased magnesium levels may precipitate hypocalcemia. Calcium and phosphorus have a reciprocal relationship: as one goes up, the other tends to go down. Hypomagnesemia may cause hypocalcemia owing to the decreased action of parathyroid hormone.

Assessment

1. **Signs and symptoms:** Numbness with tingling of fingers and circumoral region, hyperactive reflexes, muscle cramps, tetany, convulsions. Lethargy and poor feeding may be present in the newborn. In chronic hypocalcemia, fractures may be present due to bone porosity.
2. **Physical assessment:**
   - *Positive Trousseau's sign:* Ischemia-induced carpal spasm. It is elicited by applying a BP cuff to the upper arm and inflating it past systolic BP for 2 minutes.
   - *Positive Chvostek's sign:* Unilateral contraction of facial and eyelid muscles. It is elicited by irritating the facial nerve by percussing the face just in front of the ear.
3. **ECG changes:** Prolonged QT interval caused by elongation of ST segment; may develop a form of ventricular tachycardia: Torsades de pointes.

4. **History and risk factors:**
   - *Decreased ionized calcium:* For example, that occurring with alkalosis, administration of large quantities of citrated blood (citrate added to the blood to prevent clotting may bind with calcium, causing hypocalcemia), hemodilution (e.g., due to volume replacement with normal saline after hemorrhage).
   - *Increased calcium loss in body fluids:* For example, with certain diuretics.
   - *Decreased intestinal absorption:* For example, with decreased intake, impaired vitamin D metabolism (e.g., in renal failure), chronic diarrhea, post-gastrectomy.
   - *Hypoparathyroidism:* Congenital or acquired.
   - *Hyperphosphatemia:* For example, in renal failure.
   - *Hypomagnesemia.*
   - *Acute pancreatitis.*
   - *Chronic alcoholism.*

Diagnostic Tests

1. **Total serum calcium level:** May be <8.5 mg/dl. Serum calcium levels should be evaluated with serum albumin. For every 1.0 g/dl drop in the serum albumin level, there is a 0.8-1.0 mg/dl drop in total calcium level.
2. **Ionized serum calcium:** Will be <4.5 mg/dl.
3. **Parathyroid hormone:** Decreased levels occur in hypoparathyroidism; increased levels may occur with other causes of hypocalcemia. Normal range is 150-350 pg/ml (varies among laboratories).
4. **Magnesium and phosphorus levels:** May be checked to identify potential causes of hypocalcemia.

Collaborative Management

1. **Treatment of underlying cause.**
2. **Calcium replacement:** Hypocalcemia is treated with PO or IV calcium. Tetany in the adult is treated with 10-20 ml of 10% calcium gluconate IV or a continuous drip of 100 ml of 10% calcium gluconate in 1000 ml D_5W, infused over at least 4 hours.

3. **Vitamin D therapy (e.g., dihydrotachysterol, calcitriol):** To increase calcium absorption from the GI tract. See Table 9-1 for a list of vitamin D preparations.
4. **Aluminum hydroxide antacids:** To reduce elevated phosphorus level prior to treating hypocalcemia.
5. **Increased dietary intake of calcium:** At least 1000-1500 mg/day in the adult.

Nursing Diagnoses and Interventions

High risk for trauma related to potential for tetany and seizures secondary to severe hypocalcemia

Desired outcomes: Patient does not exhibit evidence of injury caused by complications of severe hypocalcemia. Serum calcium levels are within normal range (8.5-10.5 mg/dl).

1. Monitor patient for evidence of worsening hypocalcemia: numbness and tingling of fingers and circumoral region, hyperactive reflexes, and muscle cramps. Notify MD promptly if these symptoms develop because they occur prior to overt tetany. In addition, notify MD if patient has positive Trousseau's or Chvostek's signs, as they also signal latent tetany.
2. Administer IV calcium with caution. IV calcium should not be given faster than 0.5-1 ml/minute because rapid administration can cause hypotension. Observe IV insertion site for evidence of infiltration because calcium will slough tissue. Concentrated calcium solutions should be administered through a central line. Do not add calcium to solutions containing bicarbonate or phosphate because precipitates will form. Monitor patient for signs and symptoms of hypercalcemia: lethargy, confusion, irritability, nausea,

Table 9-1   Vitamin D preparations

Generic Name	Trade Name	Chemical Abbreviation
Ergocalciferol	Calciferol	D_2
Dihydrotachysterol	Hytakerol	DHT
Calcifediol	Calderol	$25(OH)D_3$
Calcitriol	Rocaltrol	$1,25(OH)_2D_3$

and vomiting. **Note:** Always clarify type of IV calcium to be given. Both calcium chloride and calcium gluconate come in 10 ml ampules. One amp of calcium chloride contains approximately 13.6 mEq of calcium, whereas one amp of calcium gluconate contains 4.5 mEq of calcium. **Note:** Digitalis toxicity may develop in patients taking digitalis because calcium potentiates its effects.

3. For patients with chronic hypocalcemia, administer oral calcium supplements and vitamin D preparations (see Table 9-1) as prescribed. Administer oral calcium 30 minutes before meals and/or at bedtime for maximal absorption. Administer aluminum hydroxide antacids immediately after meals.
4. Encourage intake of foods high in calcium: milk products, meats, leafy green vegetables (Table 9-2).
5. Notify physician if response to calcium therapy is ineffective. Tetany that does not respond to IV calcium may be caused by hypomagnesemia.
6. Keep symptomatic patients on seizure precautions; decrease environmental stimuli.
7. Avoid hyperventilation in patients in whom hypocalcemia is suspected. Respiratory alkalosis may precipitate tetany due to increased calcium-bicarbonate binding.

Decreased cardiac output related to decreased cardiac contractility secondary to hypocalcemia or digitalis toxicity occurring with calcium replacement therapy

Table 9-2 Foods high in calcium content

Cottage cheese	Seafood, especially canned sardines and canned salmon
Cheese	
Milk and cream	Rhubarb
Eggnog	Brazil nuts
Yogurt	Sesame seeds
Soy flour	Broccoli
Oat flakes	Collard, mustard, and turnip greens
Milk chocolate	
Ice cream	Spinach
Molasses	Tofu

Desired outcomes: Patient's cardiac output is adequate as evidenced by CVP ≤6 mm Hg (≤12 cm H_2O), HR ≤100, BP within patient's normal range, and absence of the clinical signs of heart failure or pulmonary edema (e.g., crackles, SOB). Critical care patients exhibit a PAP of 20-30/8-15 mm Hg.

1. Monitor ECG for signs of worsening hypocalcemia (prolonged QT interval) or digitalis toxicity with calcium replacement: multifocal or bigeminal premature ventricular contractions (PVC), paroxysmal atrial tachycardia with varying atrioventricular (AV) block, Wenckebach (Type I AV) heart block.

2. Hypocalcemia may decrease cardiac contractility. Monitor patient for signs of heart failure or pulmonary edema: crackles (rales), rhonchi, SOB, decreased BP, increased HR, increased PAP, or increased CVP.

Impaired gas exchange related to altered oxygen supply secondary to laryngeal spasm occurring with severe hypocalcemia
Desired outcome: Patient exhibits respiratory depth, pattern, and rate (12-20 breaths/min) within normal range and is asymptomatic of laryngeal spasm: laryngeal stridor, dyspnea, or crowing.

1. Assess patient's respiratory rate, character, and rhythm. Be alert to laryngeal stridor, dyspnea, and crowing, which occur with laryngeal spasm, a life-threatening complication of hypocalcemia.

2. Keep an emergency tracheostomy tray at the bedside of symptomatic patients.

Patient-Family Teaching Guidelines

Give patient and significant others verbal and written instructions for the following:

1. Medications, including drug name, purpose, dosage, frequency, precautions, and potential side effects.

2. Indicators of hypercalcemia and hypocalcemia. Review the symptoms that necessitate immediate medical attention: numbness and tingling of fingers and circumoral region and muscle cramps.

3. Foods that are high in calcium (see Table 9-1). **Note:** Many foods that are high in calcium, such as milk products, also are high in phosphorus and may need to be lim-

ited in patients with renal failure. In renal failure, a program of phosphorus control and calcium supplementation may be necessary.

Hypercalcemia

Symptomatic hypercalcemia can occur because of an increase in total serum calcium or an increase in the percentage of free, ionized calcium. If hypercalcemia is accompanied by a normal or elevated serum phosphorus level, calcium phosphate crystals may precipitate in the serum and deposit throughout the body. Soft tissue calcifications usually occur when the product (i.e., calcium × phosphorus) of the serum calcium and serum phosphorus exceeds 70 mg/dl.

 ## Assessment

1. **Signs and symptoms:** Lethargy, weakness, anorexia, nausea, vomiting, polyuria, itching, bone pain, fractures, flank pain (secondary to renal calculi), depression, confusion, paresthesias, personality changes, stupor, coma.
2. **Electrocardiogram (ECG) findings:** Shortening of ST segment and QT interval. PR interval is sometimes prolonged. Ventricular dysrhythmias can occur with severe hypercalcemia.
3. **History and risk factors:**
   - *Increased intake of calcium:* For example, excessive administration during cardiopulmonary arrest.
   - *Increased intestinal absorption:* For example, with vitamin D or A overdose or hyperparathyroidism.
   - *Increased release of calcium from bone:* Occurs with hyperparathyroidism, malignancies, prolonged immobilization, Paget's disease, hyperthyroidism.
   - *Decreased urinary excretion:* For example, renal failure, certain medications (e.g., thiazide diuretics).
   - *Increased ionized calcium:* Acidosis.

Diagnostic Tests

1. **Total serum calcium level:** May be >10.5 mg/dl.
2. **Ionized calcium:** Will be >5.5 mg/dl.

3. **Parathyroid hormone:** Increased levels occur in primary or secondary hyperparathyroidism.
4. **X-ray findings:** May reveal presence of osteoporosis, bone cavitation, or urinary calculi.

Collaborative Management

1. **Treatment of underlying cause:** For example, antitumor chemotherapy for malignancy or partial parathyroidectomy for hyperparathyroidism.
2. **IV normal saline:** Administered rapidly to increase urinary calcium excretion. Furosemide is administered to prevent fluid overload and increase calcium excretion.
3. **IV phosphates:** To cause a reciprocal drop in serum calcium.
4. **Low-calcium diet and cortisone:** To reduce intestinal absorption of calcium. Steroids compete with vitamin D, thereby reducing intestinal absorption of calcium. For a list of foods high in calcium content, see Table 9-2.
5. **Decreased bone resorption:** Accomplished *via* increased activity level, indomethacin, or mithramycin. Mithramycin, a cytotoxic antibiotic, acts directly on bone to reduce decalcification and is used primarily to treat hypercalcemia associated with neoplastic disease. Compressional loads (e.g., weight bearing) stimulate bone deposition, thus increased activity decreases bone resorption.
6. **Calcitonin:** To reduce bone resorption, increase bone deposition of calcium and phosphorus, and increase urinary calcium and phosphate excretion. Skin testing for allergy may be necessary before administration of salmon calcitonin.
7. **Hemodialysis:** Against a low calcium dialysate; used when hypercalcemia is associated with renal failure.

Nursing Diagnoses and Interventions

ndx:

High risk for injury related to neuromuscular, sensorium, or cardiac changes secondary to hypercalcemia

Desired outcomes: Patient does not exhibit evidence of injury due to neuromuscular or sensorium changes. Patient verbalizes orientation to person, place, and time. Serum calcium levels are within normal range (8.5-10.5 mg/dl).

1. Monitor patient for worsening hypercalcemia. Assess and document level of consciousness (LOC); patient's orientation to person, place, and time; and neurologic status with each vital sign (VS) check.

2. Personality changes, hallucinations, paranoia, and memory loss may occur with hypercalcemia. Inform patient and significant others that altered sensorium is temporary and will improve with treatment. Use reality therapy: clocks, calendars, and familiar objects; keep them at the bedside within patient's visual field.

3. Hypercalcemia causes neuromuscular depression with poor coordination, weakness, and altered gait. Provide a safe environment. Keep side rails up and bed in lowest position with wheels locked. Assist patient with ambulation if it is allowed.

4. Because hypercalcemia potentiates the effects of digitalis, monitor patient taking digitalis for signs and symptoms of digitalis toxicity: anorexia, nausea, vomiting, irregular pulse. ECG changes may include multifocal or bigeminal PVCs, paroxysmal atrial tachycardia with varying AV block, Wenckebach (Type 1 AV) heart block. Monitor for pulse changes in the non-ECG monitored setting.

5. Monitor serum electrolyte values for changes in serum calcium (normal range is 8.5-10.5 mg/dl); potassium (normal range is 3.5-5.0 mEq/L); and phosphorus (normal range is 2.5-4.5 mg/dl) secondary to therapy. Notify MD of abnormal values.

6. Encourage increased mobility to reduce bone resorption. Ideally, patient should be out of bed and up in a chair at least 6 hrs/day.

7. Avoid vitamin D preparations (see Table 9-1) as they increase intestinal absorption of calcium.

Altered pattern of urinary elimination related to dysuria, urgency, frequency, and polyuria secondary to administration of diuretics, calcium stone formation, or changes in renal function occurring with hypercalcemia
Desired outcome: Patient exhibits voiding pattern and urine characteristics that are normal for patient.

1. Monitor I&O hourly. Alert MD to unusual changes in urine volume, for example, oliguria alternating with poly-

uria, which may signal urinary tract obstruction, or to continuous polyuria, which may be indicative of nephrogenic diabetes insipidus.

2. Because hypercalcemia can impair renal function, monitor patient's renal function carefully: urine output, blood urea nitrogen (BUN), creatinine.
3. Provide patient with a low-calcium diet and avoid use of calcium-containing medications (e.g., antacids such as Tums).
4. Assess patient for indicators of kidney stone formation: intermittent pain, nausea, vomiting, hematuria. Encourage intake of fruits (e.g., cranberries, prunes, or plums) that leave an acid ash in the urine. An acidic urine reduces the risk of calcium stone formation.
5. Hypercalcemia leads to an increase in calcium in the urine, which inhibits the kidneys' ability to concentrate urine (nephrogenic diabetes inspidus). This leads to polyuria and potential volume depletion. Be alert to polyuria. Also monitor for signs of volume depletion when giving diuretics: decreased BP, CVP, PAP; increased HR.

Patient-Family Teaching Guidelines

Give patient and significant others verbal and written instructions for the following:

1. Medications, including drug name, purpose, dosage, frequency, precautions, and potential side effects.
2. Signs and symptoms of hypercalcemia.
3. Foods and over-the-counter (OTC) medications (e.g., antacids) that are high in calcium. See Table 9-2 for a list of foods high in calcium content. Also instruct patients to avoid vitamin supplements containing vitamins D and A.
4. If stone formation is a concern, foods that leave an acid ash in the urine. Review signs and symptoms of nephrolithiasis.
5. After hospital discharge, the importance of increased fluid intake (up to 4 L in nonrestricted patients) to minimize risk of stone formation.

Disorders of Phosphorus Balance

10

Phosphorus is the primary anion of the intracellular fluid (ICF). Approximately 85% of the body's phosphorus is located in the bones and teeth, 14% is in the soft tissue, and less than 1% is within the extracellular fluid (ECF). Because of the large intracellular store, under certain acute conditions, phosphorus may move into or out of the cell, causing dramatic changes in plasma phosphorus. Chronically, substantial increases or decreases can occur in intracellular phosphorus levels without significantly altering plasma levels. Thus, plasma phosphorus levels do not necessarily reflect intracellular levels. Although most laboratories measure and report elemental phosphorus, nearly all the phosphorus in the body exists in the form of phosphate (PO_4^{3-}) and the terms phosphorus and phosphate often are used interchangeably.

Phosphorus is an important constituent of all body tissues and has a wide variety of vital functions, including formation of energy storing substances (e.g., adenosine triphosphate [ATP]); formation of red blood cell 2,3-diphosphoglycerate (DPG), which facilitates oxygen delivery to the tissues; metabolism of carbohydrates, protein, and fat; and maintenance of acid-base balance. In addition, phosphorus is critical to normal nerve and muscle function and provides structural support to bones and teeth. Plasma PO_4^{3-} levels vary with age, gender, and diet. Levels decrease with increasing age, with the exception of a slight rise in PO_4^{3-} in women following menopause. Glucose, insulin, or sugar-containing foods cause a temporary drop in PO_4^{3-} due to a shift of serum PO_4^{3-} into the cells.

Acid-base status also will affect phosphorus balance. Alkalosis, particularly respiratory alkalosis, may cause hypophosphatemia owing to an intracellular shift of phosphorus. The exact mechanism for this shift is not fully understood but may be related to an alkalosis-induced cellular glycolysis with increased formation of phosphorus-containing metabolic intermediates. Respiratory acidosis may cause a shift of phosphorus out of the cells and contribute to hyperphosphatemia.

The level of ECF phosphate is regulated by a combination of factors, including dietary intake, intestinal absorption, renal excretion, and hormonally regulated bone resorption and deposition. Phosphorus balance is closely tied to that of calcium. Normal range for serum phosphorus is 2.5-4.5 mg/dl (1.7-2.6 mEq/L).

Hypophosphatemia

Hypophosphatemia (serum phosphorus <2.5 mg/dl) may occur due to transient intracellular shifts, increased urinary losses, decreased intestinal absorption, or increased utilization (see "History and Risk Factors", in the following section). Severe phosphorus deficiency also may occur with alcoholism, especially during acute withdrawal, owing to poor intake, vomiting and diarrhea, hyperventilation, use of phosphorus-binding antacids, and increased urinary losses. In addition, a combination of factors may lead to hypophosphatemia in diabetic ketoacidosis (DKA). In DKA there is a significant loss of phosphorus in the urine secondary to the glucose-induced osmotic diuresis. This developing hypophosphatemia is masked, however, by the movement of phosphorus out of the cells due to increased tissue catabolism (cellular breakdown). When ketoacidosis is treated with glucose, insulin, and fluids, there is a dramatic shift of phosphorus back into the cells and the existing phosphorus depletion then becomes apparent. For more information about DKA see Chapter 20.

Assessment

1. **Signs and symptoms:** Patients may present with acute symptoms due to sudden decreases in serum phosphorus, or symptoms may develop gradually owing to chronic phosphorus deficiency. The majority of symptoms are secondary to decreases in ATP and 2,3-DPG.

- *Acute:* Confusion, seizures, coma, chest pain due to poor oxygenation of the myocardium, muscle pain, increased susceptibility to infection, numbness and tingling of the fingers and circumoral region, and incoordination.
- *Chronic:* Memory loss, lethargy, bone pain.

2. **Physical assessment:**
   - *Acute:* Decreased strength as evidenced by difficulty speaking, weakness of respiratory muscles, and weakening hand grasp. Hypoxia may cause an increased respiratory rate (RR) and respiratory alkalosis (secondary to hyperventilation). **Note:** Respiratory alkalosis causes phosphorus to move intracellularly, aggravating the existing hypophosphatemia.
   - *Chronic:* Bruising and bleeding may occur due to platelet dysfunction. Lethargy, weakness, joint stiffness, arthralgia, osteomalacia, cyanosis, and pseudofractures may occur.

3. **Hemodynamic measurements:** Severely depleted patients may show signs of decreased myocardial function, including increased pulmonary artery wedge pressure (PAWP), decreased cardiac output (CO), and decreased blood pressure (BP) with decreased response to pressor agents.

4. **History and risk factors:**
   - *Intracellular shifts:* Carbohydrate load; respiratory alkalosis (see Chapter 14); nutritional recovery (usually associated with TPN); androgen therapy; recovery from burns.
   - *Increased utilization due to increased tissue repair:* Total parenteral nutrition with inadequate phosphorus content; recovery from protein-calorie malnutrition.
   - *Increased urinary losses:* Hypomagnesemia (see Chapter 11); hypokalemia; hyperparathyroidism; use of thiazide diuretics; familial hypophosphatemic rickets; Fanconi's syndrome.
   - *Reduced intestinal absorption or increased intestinal loss:* Use of phosphorus-binding antacids (e.g., aluminum hydroxide antacids such as Amphojel or Alternajel); vomiting and diarrhea; malabsorption disorders such as vitamin D deficiency.
   - *Mixed causes:* Alcoholism, DKA (with treatment), severe burns.

Diagnostic Tests

1. **Serum phosphorus:** Will be <2.5 mg/dl (1.7 mEq/L).
   - *Moderate hypophosphatemia:* <1.0-2.5 mg/dl.
   - *Severe hypophosphatemia:* <1.0 mg/dl.
2. **Parathyroid hormone (PTH) level:** Will be elevated in hyperparathyroidism.
3. **Serum magnesium:** May be decreased owing to increased urinary excretion of magnesium in hypophosphatemia.
4. **Alkaline phosphatase:** Increased with increased osteoblastic activity.
5. **X-rays:** May reveal skeletal changes of osteomalacia or rickets.

Collaborative Management

1. **Identification and elimination of the cause:** For example, avoiding use of phosphorus-binding antacids (aluminum, magnesium, or calcium gels or antacids).
2. **Phosphorus supplementation:** Mild hypophosphatemia may be treated by increasing intake of high-phosphorus foods (Table 10-1). Mild to moderate hypophosphatemia usually can be treated with oral phosphate supplements such as Neutra Phor (sodium and potassium phosphate) or Phospho-Soda (sodium phosphate). IV sodium phosphate or potassium phosphate is necessary in cases of severe hypophosphatemia or when the GI tract is nonfunctional.

Table 10-1   Foods high in phosphorus

Meats, especially organ meats (e.g., brain, liver, kidney)
Fish
Poultry
Milk and milk products (e.g., cheese, ice cream, cottage cheese)
Whole grains (e.g., oatmeal, bran, barley)
Seeds (e.g., pumpkin, sesame, sunflower)
Nuts (e.g., Brazil, peanuts)
Eggs and egg products (e.g., egg nog, souffles)
Dried beans and peas

Nursing Diagnoses and Interventions

High risk for injury related to sensory or neuromuscular dysfunction secondary to hypophosphatemia-induced central nervous system (CNS) disturbances

Desired outcome: Patient verbalizes orientation to person, place, and time and does not exhibit evidence of injury due to altered sensorium.

1. Monitor serum phosphorus levels in patients at increased risk. Notify MD of decreased levels.

2. Apprehension, confusion, and paresthesias are signals of developing hypophosphatemia. Assess and document level of consciousness (LOC), orientation, and neurologic status with each vital sign check. Reorient patient as necessary. Alert MD to significant changes.

3. Inform patient and significant others that altered sensorium is temporary and will improve with treatment.

4. Do not administer IV phosphate at a rate greater than that recommended by the manufacturer. Potential complications of IV phosphorus administration include *tetany,* owing to hypocalcemia (serum calcium levels may drop suddenly if serum phosphorus levels increase suddenly—see Chapter 9, pp. 109–111 for additional information); *soft tissue calcification* (if the patient develops hyperphosphatemia, the calcium and phosphorus in the ECF may combine and form deposits in tissue—see discussion p. 125; and *hypotension,* caused by a too rapid delivery. When IV phosphorus is administered as potassium phosphate, the infusion rate should not exceed 10 mEq/hr. Monitor the IV site for signs of infiltration, as potassium phosphate can cause necrosis and sloughing of tissue (see Chapter 8, p. 99, for precautions when administering IV potassium).

5. Keep the side rails up and the bed in its lowest position, with wheels locked.

6. Use reality therapy, such as clocks, calendars, and familiar objects. Keep these articles at the bedside, within patient's visual field.

7. If patient is at risk for seizures, pad the side rails and keep an airway at the bedside.

Impaired gas exchange related to altered oxygen supply to the tissues secondary to decreased strength of respiratory muscles, decreased cardiac function, and decreased 2,3-DPG

Note: With decreased 2,3-DPG levels, the oxyhemoglobin dissociation curve will shift to the right. That is, at a given oxygen tension of arterial blood (Pao_2) level, more oxygen will be bound to hemoglobin and less will be available to the tissues.

Desired outcome: Patient exhibits normal respiratory function as evidenced by RR 12-20 breaths/min with normal depth and pattern (eupnea); normal skin color; absence of chest pain; and orientation to person, place, and time.

1. Monitor rate and depth of respirations in patients who are severely hypophosphatemic. Alert MD to changes.
2. Assess patient for signs of hypoxia: restlessness, confusion, increased RR, complaints of chest pain, and cyanosis (a late sign).
3. Also see interventions for **Decreased cardiac output,** below.

Impaired physical mobility (or risk of same) related to osteomalacia with bone pain and fractures owing to movement of phosphorus out of the bone secondary to chronic hypophosphatemia; or muscle weakness and acute rhabdomyolysis (breakdown of striated muscle) secondary to severe hypophosphatemia

Desired outcome: Patient has mobility without evidence of weakness, pain, or fractures.

1. Monitor all patients with suspected hypophosphatemia for evidence of decreasing muscle strength. Perform serial assessments of hand grasp strength and clarity of speech. Alert MD to changes.
2. Monitor serum phosphorus levels for evidence of worsening hypophosphatemia. Alert MD to changes.
3. Assist the patient with ambulation and with activities of daily living (ADL). Keep personal items within easy reach.
4. Encourage the intake of foods high in phosphorus. See Table 10-1.
5. Medicate for pain as prescribed.

Decreased cardiac output related to negative inotropic changes associated with reduced myocardial functioning secondary to severe phosphorus depletion

Desired outcomes: Patient's cardiac output is adequate as evidenced by CVP <6 mm Hg, HR ≤100 bpm, BP within patient's normal range, and absence of the clinical signs of heart failure or pulmonary edema. Critical care patients exhibit PAP 20-30/8-15 mm Hg.

1. Monitor patient for signs of heart failure or pulmonary edema: crackles (rales), rhonchi, shortness of breath (SOB), decreased BP, increased HR, increased PAP, or increased CVP.
2. Prevent patient from hyperventilating, if possible, as respiratory alkalosis will cause an increased movement of phosphorus into the cells.

High risk for infection related to impaired white blood cell (WBC) functioning secondary to reduced ATP
Desired outcome: Patient is free of infection as evidenced by afebrile state and absence of erythema, swelling, warmth, and purulent drainage at invasive sites.

1. Monitor temperature and secretions every 4 hours for evidence of infection. Culture suspicious secretions as prescribed.
2. Use meticulous, aseptic technique when changing dressings or manipulating indwelling lines (e.g., total parenteral nutrition catheters, IV needles).
3. Provide oral hygiene and skin care at regular intervals. Intact skin and membranes are the body's first line of defense against infection.

 Patient-Family Teaching Guidelines

Give patient and significant others verbal and written instructions for the following:

1. Medications, including drug name, purpose, dosage, frequency, precautions, and potential side effects.
2. Indicators of hypophosphatemia and hyperphosphatemia. Review the symptoms that necessitate immediate medical attention: weakness, SOB, numbness and tingling of fingers and circumoral region. For patients at risk for chronic hypophosphatemia, alert them to the need for notifying MD of the presence of bone pain.

3. Foods that are high in phosphorus, if a high phosphorus diet is encouraged (see Table 10-1).

4. Importance of using phosphorus-binding antacids *only* as prescribed by physician.

Hyperphosphatemia

Hyperphosphatemia occurs most often in the presence of renal insufficiency due to the kidneys' decreased ability to excrete excess phosphorus. In addition to renal failure, other causes of hyperphosphatemia include increased intake of phosphates, extra-cellular shifts (i.e., movement of phosphorus out of the cell and into the ECF), cellular destruction with concomitant release of intracellular phosphorus, and decreased urinary losses that are unrelated to decreased renal function. As serum phosphorus levels increase, serum calcium levels often drop, which may cause hypocalcemia to develop (see Chapter 9 for additional information). Hypocalcemia is most likely to occur in sudden, severe hyperphosphatemia (e.g., after IV administration of phosphates) or when the patient already is prone to hypocalcemia (e.g., with chronic renal failure).

The primary complication of hyperphosphatemia is metastatic calcification (i.e., the precipitation of calcium phosphate in the soft tissue, joints, and arteries). Precipitation of calcium phosphate occurs when the calcium-phosphorus product (calcium $\times$ phosphorus) exceeds 70 mg/dl. Chronic hyperphosphatemia in the patient with chronic renal failure may contribute to the development of renal osteodystrophy.

Assessment

1. **Signs and symptoms:** Anorexia, nausea, vomiting, muscle weakness, hyperreflexia, tetany, tachycardia. **Note:** Usually, patients experience few symptoms with hyperphosphatemia. The majority of symptoms that do occur relate to the development of hypocalcemia or soft tissue (metastatic) calcifications. Indicators of metastatic calcification include oliguria, corneal haziness, conjunctivitis, irregular heart rate, and papular eruptions.

2. **Physical assessment:** See "Hypocalcemia," p. 109. In addition, see "Signs and Symptoms," p. 125, for indicators of metastatic calcifications.
3. **ECG changes:** See "Hypocalcemia," p. 109. Deposition of calcium phosphate in the heart may lead to dysrhythmias and conduction disturbances.
4. **History and risk factors:**
   - *Renal failure:* Acute and chronic.
   - *Increased intake:* Excessive administration of phosphorus supplements; vitamin D excess with increased GI absorption; excessive use of phosphorus-containing laxatives or enemas (especially in children).
   - *Extracellular shift:* Respiratory acidosis; diabetic ketoacidosis (prior to treatment).
   - *Cellular destruction:* Neoplastic disease (e.g., leukemia and lymphoma) treated with cytotoxic agents; increased tissue catabolism (breakdown); rhabdomyolysis (breakdown of striated muscle).
   - *Decreased urinary losses:* Hypoparathyroidism; volume depletion.

Diagnostic Tests

1. **Serum phosphorus:** Will be >4.5 mg/dl (2.6 mEq/L).
   Note: Improper handling of blood specimens may result in factitious (false) hyperphosphatemia due to hemolysis of blood cells.
2. **Serum calcium level:** Useful in assessing potential consequences of treatment and diagnosis of primary problem.
3. **X-ray:** May show skeletal changes of osteodystrophy.
4. **Parathyroid hormone:** Level will be decreased in hypoparathyroidism.
5. **Blood urea nitrogen (BUN) and creatinine:** To assess renal function.

Collaborative Management

1. **Identification and elimination of the cause** (e.g., correction of volume depletion).
2. **Use of aluminum, magnesium, or calcium gels or ant-**

acids: To bind phosphorus in the gut, thus increasing GI elimination of phosphorus. **Note:** Magnesium antacids are avoided in renal failure due to the risk of hypermagnesemia. Serum phosphorus levels may be allowed to remain slightly elevated (4.5-6.0 mg/dl) in chronic renal failure to ensure adequate levels of 2,3-DPG. This helps to limit the effects of chronic anemia on oxygen delivery to the tissues.

3. **Diet low in phosphorus:** See Table 10-1 for a list of foods that should be avoided.
4. **Dialytic therapy:** May be necessary for acute, severe hyperphosphatemia accompanied by symptomatic hypocalcemia.

Nursing Diagnoses and Interventions

Knowledge deficit: Purpose of phosphate binders and the importance of reducing gastrointestinal absorption of phosphorus to control hyperphosphatemia and prevent long-term complications **Desired outcome:** Patient describes the potential complications of uncontrolled hyperphosphatemia and the ways in which they can be prevented. **Note:** Because symptoms of hyperphosphatemia may be minimal, the prevention of long-term complications relies primarily on adequate patient education.

1. Teach patients the purpose of phosphate binders. Stress the need to take binders as prescribed with or after meals to maximize effectiveness.
2. Prepare patients for the possibility of constipation secondary to binder use. Encourage use of bulk-building supplements or stool softener if constipation occurs. Phosphate-containing laxatives and enemas must be avoided.
3. Phosphate binders are available in liquid or capsule form. Confer with MD regarding an alternate form or brand for individuals who find binders unpalatable or difficult to take. Phosphate binders vary in their aluminum, magnesium, or calcium content, however, and one may not be exchanged for another without first ensuring that the patient is receiving the same amount of elemental aluminum, magnesium, or calcium.
4. Encourage patient to avoid or limit foods high in phosphorus. (See Table 10-1.)

High risk for injury related to precipitation of calcium phosphate in the soft tissue (e.g., cornea, lungs, kidney, gastric mucosa, heart, blood vessels) and periarticular region of the large joints (e.g., hips, shoulders, and elbows) or development of hypocalcemic tetany

Desired outcomes: Patient exhibits no evidence of metastatic calcification or hypocalcemia. The calcium-phosphorus product (calcium × phosphorus) remains <70 mg/dl.

1. Monitor serum phosphorus and calcium levels. Alert MD to abnormal values. Remember that phosphorus values may be kept slightly higher (4.5-6.0 mg/dl) in chronic renal failure patients to ensure adequate levels of 2,3-DPG, thereby minimizing effects of chronic anemia on oxygen delivery to the tissues.

2. Avoid vitamin D products (see Table 9-1) and calcium supplements until the serum phosphorus level approaches normal.

3. Alert MD to indicators of metastatic calcification: oliguria, corneal haziness, conjunctivitis, irregular heart rate, and papular eruptions.

4. Monitor patient for evidence of increasing hypocalcemia: numbness and tingling of the fingers and circumoral region, hyperactive reflexes, and muscle cramps. Notify MD promptly if these symptoms develop because they occur prior to overt tetany. In addition, alert MD if patient has positive Trousseau's or Chvostek's signs, as they signal latent tetany (see Chapter 4, p. 35, for a discussion of these signs and Chapter 9 for additional information regarding treatment and prevention of hypocalcemia).

5. Because hyperphosphatemia can impair renal function, monitor patient's renal function carefully: urine output, BUN, and creatinine. For additional information, see "Acute Renal Failure," p. 218.

Patient-Family Teaching Guidelines

Give patient and significant others verbal and written instructions for the following:

1. Medications, including drug name, purpose, dosage, frequency, precautions, and potential side effects.

2. Indicators of hyperphosphatemia and hypocalcemia. Review the symptoms that require immediate medical attention: weakness, SOB, and numbness and tingling of fingers and circumoral region. For patients with chronic hyperphosphatemia, alert them to the necessity of notifying MD if symptoms of metastatic calcification occur.

3. Foods that are high in phosphorus and thus, must be avoided (see Table 10-1).

4. Importance of avoiding phosphorus-containing over-the-counter medications: certain laxatives, enemas, and multivitamin and mineral supplements. Instruct patient and significant others to read labels for the words "phosphorus" and "phosphate."

Disorders of Magnesium Balance 11

Magnesium is the body's fourth most abundant cation, yet its measurement and evaluation often are overlooked. Of the body's magnesium, approximately 50-60% is located in bone and approximately 1% is located in the extracellular fluid (ECF). The remaining magnesium is contained within the cells, thereby constituting the second most abundant intracellular cation after potassium. Magnesium is regulated by a combination of factors, including vitamin D-controlled gastrointestinal absorption and renal excretion. Normally, only about 30-40% of dietary magnesium is absorbed. Renal excretion of magnesium changes to maintain magnesium balance and is affected by sodium and calcium excretion, ECF volume, and the presence of parathyroid hormone (PTH). It is decreased with increased PTH, decreased excretion of sodium or calcium, and fluid volume deficit.

Because magnesium is a major intracellular ion, it plays a vital role in normal cellular function. Specifically, it activates enzymes involved in the metabolism of carbohydrates and protein, and triggers the sodium-potassium pump, thus affecting intracellular potassium levels. Magnesium also is important in the transmission of neuromuscular activity, neural transmission within the central nervous system (CNS), and myocardial functioning.

Normal serum magnesium level is 1.5-2.5 mEq/L. Approximately one quarter to one third of the plasma magnesium is bound to protein, a small portion is combined with other substances (complexed), and the remaining portion is free or ionized. It is the free ionized magnesium that is physiologically important. As with calcium levels, magnesium levels should be evaluated in combination with serum albumin levels. Low serum albumin levels will decrease the total magnesium level, whereas the amount of free ionized magnesium may be unchanged.

Hypomagnesemia

Hypomagnesemia (serum magnesium level <1.5 mEq/L) usually occurs because of decreased GI absorption or increased urinary loss. It also may occur with excessive GI loss (e.g., vomiting, diarrhea) or with prolonged administration of magnesium-free parenteral fluids. Alcoholics (see **History and risk factors,** below) and critical care patients are the two most common patient populations. Hypomagnesemia usually is associated with hypocalcemia and hypokalemia (see "Diagnostic Tests," p. 132 for additional information). Symptoms of hypomagnesemia tend to develop once the serum magnesium level drops below 1 mEq/L.

Assessment

1. **Signs and symptoms:** Apathy, leg cramps, insomnia, mood changes, hallucinations, confusion, anorexia, nausea, vomiting, paresthesias.
2. **Physical assessment:** Increased reflexes, tremors, convulsions, tetany, and positive Chvostek's and Trousseau's signs (see Chapter 4, p. 109) in part owing to accompanying hypocalcemia. The patient also may have tachycardia and hypertension.
3. **Hemodynamic measurements:** See "Hypocalcemia," p. 109 and "Hypokalemia," p. 98.
4. **History and risk factors:**
   - *Chronic alcoholism:* A common cause of hypomagnesemia due to a combination of poor dietary intake, decreased GI absorption, and increased urinary excretion secondary to ethanol effect.
   - *Malabsorption syndrome:* For example, due to cancer, colitis, pancreatic insufficiency, surgical resection of the GI tract.
   - *Vomiting, NG suction, diarrhea.*
   - *Administration of low-magnesium or magnesium-free parenteral solutions.*
   - *Protein-calorie malnutrition.*

- *Hyperaldosteronism:* Due to volume expansion.
- *Diabetic ketoacidosis:* Owing to movement of magnesium out of the cell and loss in the urine because of osmotic diuresis secondary to glucosuria.
- *Drugs that enhance urinary excretion:* For example, diuretics, amphotericin, tobramycin, gentamicin, cisplatin, digoxin, cyclosporine.

Diagnostic Tests

1. **Serum magnesium level:** Will be less than 1.5 mEq/L. Unfortunately, a normal serum magnesium level does not eliminate the possibility of an intracellular deficiency.
2. **Urinary magnesium level:** Helps identify renal causes of magnesium depletion; may be performed after parenteral administration of magnesium sulfate (magnesium loading test).
3. **Serum albumin level:** A decreased albumin level may cause a decreased magnesium level due to a reduction in protein-bound magnesium. The amount of free ionized magnesium may be unchanged.
4. **Serum potassium level:** May be decreased owing to failure of the cellular sodium-potassium pump to move potassium into the cell and the accompanying loss of potassium in the urine. This hypokalemia may be resistant to potassium replacement until the magnesium deficit has been corrected.
5. **Serum calcium level:** Hypomagnesemia may lead to hypocalcemia due to a reduction in the release and action of parathyroid hormone (PTH). PTH is the primary regulator of serum calcium levels (see Chapter 9).
6. **ECG evaluations:** May reflect magnesium, as well as calcium and potassium deficiencies: tachyarrhythmias, prolonged PR and QT intervals, widening of the QRS, ST segment depression, and flattened T waves. A form of ventricular tachycardia (Torsades de pointes) associated with all three electrolyte imbalances may develop. Increased digitalis effect, as evidenced by multifocal or bigeminal premature ventricular contractions (PVCs), paroxysmal atrial tachycardia with varying AV block, and Wenckebach (Type I AV) heart block, also may occur.

Collaborative Management

1. **Identification and elimination of the cause:** For example, adequate replacement of magnesium in total parenteral nutrition solutions.
2. **IV or intramuscular (IM) magnesium sulfate (MgSO₄):** For severe or symptomatic hypomagnesemia.
3. **Oral magnesium:** Magnesium-containing antacids (e.g., Mylanta, Maalox, Gelusil, milk of magnesia) may be used.
4. **Increased dietary intake of magnesium:** See Table 11-1.

Nursing Diagnoses and Interventions

High risk for injury related to sensory or neuromuscular dysfunction secondary to hypomagnesemia
Desired outcomes: Patient does not exhibit evidence of injury caused by complications of severe hypomagnesemia. Serum magnesium levels are within normal range (1.5-2.5 mEq/L).

1. Monitor serum magnesium levels in patient at risk for developing hypomagnesemia, for example those who are alcoholics or receiving medications that increase urinary excretion. Alert MD to abnormal values. **Note:** Symptomatic hypomagnesemia may be mistakenly attributed to delirium tremens of chronic alcoholism. Be especially

Table 11-1 Foods high in magnesium

Green, leafy vegetables (e.g., beet greens, collard greens)
Seafood and meat
Nuts and seeds
Wheat bran
Soy flour
Milk
Legumes
Bananas
Oranges
Grapefruit
Chocolate
Molasses
Coconuts
Refined sugar

alert to indicators of magnesium deficit in these patients.

2. Administer IV MgSO$_4$ with caution. Refer to manufacturer's guidelines. Too rapid an administration may lead to dangerous hypermagnesemia with cardiac or respiratory arrest. Patients receiving IV magnesium should be monitored for decreasing BP, labored respirations, and diminished patellar (knee jerk) reflex. An absent patellar reflex is a signal of hyporeflexia due to dangerous hypermagnesemia. Should any of these changes occur, stop the infusion and notify the MD *stat* (see "Hypermagnesemia," p. 136. Keep calcium gluconate at the bedside in the event of hypocalcemic tetany or sudden hypermagnesemia.

3. For patients with chronic hypomagnesemia, administer oral magnesium supplements as prescribed. All magnesium supplements should be given with caution in patients with reduced renal function owing to an increased risk of the development of hypermagnesemia. Diarrhea is a common side effect of oral magnesium supplements. Alert MD if diarrhea develops.

4. Encourage the intake of foods high in magnesium in appropriate patients (see Table 11-1). **Note:** For most patients, a regular diet usually is adequate.

5. Keep symptomatic patients on seizure precautions. Decrease environmental stimuli (e.g., keep the room quiet, use subdued lighting).

6. For patients in whom hypocalcemia is suspected, caution against hyperventilation. Respiratory alkalosis may precipitate tetany, owing to increased calcium binding.

7. Dysphagia may occur in hypomagnesemia. Test the patient's ability to swallow water prior to giving food or medications.

8. Assess and document level of consciousness (LOC), orientation, and neurologic status with each vital sign check. Reorient patient as necessary. Alert MD to significant changes. Inform patient and significant others that altered mood and sensorium are temporary and will improve with treatment.

9. Alert MD to patients receiving magnesium-free solutions

(e.g., total parenteral nutrition) for prolonged periods of time.
10. See "Hypokalemia," pp. 98–103 and "Hypocalcemia," pp. 109–114, for nursing care of these disorders. **Note:** Because magnesium is necessary for the movement of potassium into the cell, intracellular potassium deficits cannot be corrected until hypomagnesemia has been treated effectively.

Decreased cardiac output related to electrical alterations associated with tachyarrhythmias or digitalis toxicity secondary to hypomagnesemia

Desired Outcome: Electrocardiogram (ECG) shows normal configuration and heart rate is within normal range for the patient.
1. Monitor heart rate and regularity with each VS check. Alert MD to changes.
2. Assess ECG in patient on continuous ECG monitoring.
3. Because hypomagnesemia (and hypokalemia) potentiates the cardiac effects of digitalis, monitor patients taking digitalis for digitalis-induced dysrhythmias. ECG changes may include multifocal or bigeminal PVCs, paroxysmal atrial tachycardia with varying AV block, and Wenckebach (Type I AV) heart block. Monitor for pulse changes in the non-ECG monitored setting.

Altered nutrition: Less than body requirements of magnesium related to history of poor intake or anorexia, nausea, and vomiting secondary to hypomagnesemia

Desired outcome: Patient verbalizes knowledge of foods high in magnesium content and demonstrates consumption of these foods during meals.
1. Encourage intake of small, frequent meals.
2. Teach patient about foods high in magnesium content (see Table 11-1) and encourage intake of these foods.
3. Medicate with antiemetics as prescribed.
4. Include patient, significant others, and dietitian in meal planning as appropriate.
5. Provide oral hygiene before meals to enhance appetite.

Patient-Family Teaching Guidelines

Give patient and significant others verbal and written instructions for the following:

1. Medications, including drug name, purpose, dosage, frequency, precautions, and potential side effects.
2. Indicators of hypo- and hypermagnesemia and hypocalcemia. Emphasize the symptoms that necessitate immediate medical attention: numbness and tingling of fingers and circumoral region, muscle cramps, altered sensorium, and irregular or rapid pulse.
3. Foods that are high in magnesium (see Table 11-1). Review the prescribed diet with the patient.
4. Referrals to Alcoholics Anonymous, Al-anon, and Al-ateen as appropriate for the alcoholic patient and his or her significant others.

Hypermagnesemia

Hypermagnesemia (serum magnesium levels >2.5 mEq/L) occurs almost exclusively in individuals with renal failure who have an increased intake of magnesium (e.g., use of magnesium-containing medications). It also may occur in acute adrenocortical insufficiency (Addison's disease) or during hypothermia. In rare cases, hypermagnesemia occurs because of excessive use of magnesium-containing medications (e.g., antacids, laxatives, enemas). The primary symptoms of hypermagnesemia are the result of depressed peripheral and central neuromuscular transmission. Symptoms usually do not occur until the magnesium level exceeds 4 mEq/L.

Assessment

1. **Signs and symptoms:** Nausea, vomiting, flushing, diaphoresis, sensation of heat, altered mental functioning, drowsiness, coma, and muscular weakness or paralysis. Paralysis of the respiratory muscles may occur when the magnesium level exceeds 10 mEq/L.
2. **Physical assessment:** Hypotension, soft tissue (metastatic) calcification (see description, p. 125), bradycardia, and decreased deep tendon reflexes. The patellar (knee jerk)

reflex is lost once the magnesium level exceeds 8 mEq/L.
3. **Hemodynamic measurements:** Decreased arterial pressure due to peripheral vasodilatation.
4. **History and risk factors:**
   - *Decreased excretion of magnesium:* For example, with renal failure or adrenocortical insufficiency.
   - *Increased intake of magnesium:* For example, excessive use of magnesium-containing antacids, enemas, and laxatives or excessive administration of magnesium sulfate (e.g., in the treatment of hypomagnesemia or pregnancy-induced hypertension).

Diagnostic Tests

1. **Serum magnesium level:** Will be >2.5 mEq/L.
2. **ECG findings:** Prolonged QT interval and AV block may occur in severe hypermagnesemia (levels >12 mEq/L).

Collaborative Management

1. **Removal of cause:** For example, discontinuing or avoiding use of magnesium-containing medications or supplements, especially in patients with decreased renal function. See Table 11-2 for a list of medications that contain magnesium.
2. **Diuretics and 0.45% sodium chloride solution:** To enhance magnesium excretion in patients with adequate renal function.
3. **IV calcium gluconate, 10 ml of a 10% solution:** To antagonize the neuromuscular effects of magnesium for patients with potentially lethal hypermagnesemia.
4. **Dialysis with magnesium-free dialysate:** For patients with severely decreased renal function.

Nursing Diagnoses and Interventions

High risk for injury related to altered mental functioning, drowsiness and weakness, or metastatic calcification secondary to hypermagnesemia
Desired outcomes: Patient verbalizes orientation to person, place, and time and does not exhibit evidence of injury owing to

Table 11-2 Magnesium-containing medications

Antacids

Aludrox
Camalox
Di-Gel
Gaviscon
Gelusil and Gelusil II
Maalox and Maalox Plus
Mylanta and Mylanta II
Riopan
Simeco
Tempo

Magnesium-Containing Mineral Supplements

Laxatives

Magnesium hydroxide (milk of magnesia, Haley's M-O)
Magnesium citrate
Magnesium sulfate (Epsom salts)

---

complications of hypermagnesemia. Patient is asymptomatic of soft tissue (metastatic) calcifications: oliguria, corneal haziness conjunctivitis, irregular heart rate, and papular eruptions. Serum magnesium levels are within normal range (1.5-2.5 mEq/L).

1. Monitor serum magnesium levels in the patient at risk for developing hypermagnesemia, for example, those with chronic renal failure or women being treated for pregnancy-induced hypertension.

2. Assess and document LOC, orientation, and neurologic status (e.g., hand grasp) with each VS check. Assess patellar (knee jerk) reflex in patients with a moderately elevated magnesium level (>5 mEq/L). With patient lying flat, support the knee in a moderately flexed position and tap the patellar tendon firmly just below the patella. Normally, the knee will extend. An absent reflex suggests a magnesium level of ≥7 mEq/L. Alert MD to significant changes.

3. Reassure patient and significant others that altered mental functioning and muscle strength will improve with treatment.

4. Keep side rails up and the bed in its lowest position with the wheels locked.
5. Assess patient for the development of soft tissue calcification. Notify MD of significant findings.
6. Infants born to mothers receiving parenteral magnesium should be monitored for hypermagnesemia (e.g., neurologic depression, low Apgar scores).
7. Hypermagnesemia is often treated with IV calcium because it reverses the toxic effects of excess magnesium. The effects are temporary and repeated doses may be necessary. Keep calcium at the bedside of symptomatic patients.

Knowledge deficit: Importance of avoiding excessive or inappropriate use of magnesium-containing medications, especially for patients with chronic renal failure

Desired outcome: Patient verbalizes the importance of avoiding un usual magnesium intake and identifies potential sources of unwanted magnesium.

1. Caution patients with chronic renal failure to review all over-the-counter medications with health care provider before use.
2. Provide a list of common magnesium-containing medications (see Table 11-2).
3. Patients with renal failure usually are on vitamin supplements. Caution these patients to avoid combination vitamin-mineral supplements as they usually contain magnesium.

Patient-Family Teaching Guidelines

Give patient and significant others verbal and written instructions for the following:

1. Medications, including drug name, dosage, purpose, schedule, precautions, and potential side effects.
2. Indicators of hypermagnesemia. Review symptoms that require immediate medical attention: altered mental functioning, drowsiness, and muscle weakness.
3. Magnesium-containing medications that should be avoided (see Table 11-2).

Overview of Acid-Base Balance

12

For optimal functioning of the cells, metabolic processes maintain a steady balance between acids and bases. Arterial pH is an indirect measurement of hydrogen ion (H^+) concentration (i.e., the greater the concentration, the more acidic the solution and the lower the pH; the lower the concentration, the more alkaline the solution and the higher the pH) and is a reflection of the balance between carbon dioxide (CO_2), which is regulated by the lungs, and bicarbonate (HCO_3^-), a base regulated by the kidneys. CO_2 dissolves in solution to form carbonic acid (H_2CO_3), which is the key acid component in acid-base balance. Because H_2CO_3 is difficult to measure directly and CO_2 and H_2CO_3 are in balance, the acid component is expressed as CO_2 instead of H_2CO_3.

Normal acid-base ratio is 1:20, representing one part CO_2 (potential H_2CO_3) to twenty parts HCO_3^-. If this balance is altered, derangements in pH occur: if extra acids are present or there is a loss of base and the pH is < 7.40, acidosis exists; if extra base is present or there is loss of acid and the pH is > 7.40, alkalosis is present. Several mechanisms regulate acid-base balance. These mechanisms are exceptionally sensitive to minute changes in pH and the body usually is able to maintain pH without outside intervention, if not at a normal level, at least within a life-sustaining range.

Buffer System Responses
Buffers

Buffers are present in all body fluids and act immediately (within 1 second) after an abnormal pH occurs. They combine with excess acid or base to form substances that do not affect pH. Their effect, however, is limited.

1. **Bicarbonate:** The most important buffer, it is present in the largest quantity in body fluids. It is generated by the kidneys and aids in the excretion of H^+.
2. **Phosphate:** Aids in the excretion of H^+ in the renal tubules.
3. **Ammonium:** After an acid load, ammonia (NH_3) is produced by the renal tubular cell and is combined with H^+ in the renal tubule to form ammonium (NH_4^+). This process allows greater renal excretion of H^+.
4. **Protein:** Present in cells, blood, and plasma. Hemoglobin is the most important protein buffer.

Respiratory System

Hydrogen ions exert direct action on the respiratory center in the brain. Acidemia increases alveolar ventilation to 4-5 times the normal level, whereas alkalemia decreases alveolar ventilation to 50%-75% of the normal level. The response occurs quickly— within 1-2 minutes, during which time the lungs eliminate or retain carbon dioxide in direct relation to arterial pH. Although the respiratory system cannot correct imbalances completely, it is 50%-70% effective.

Renal System

This system regulates acid-base balance by increasing or decreasing bicarbonate concentration in body fluids. This is accomplished through a series of complex reactions that involve H^+, sodium ion (Na^+), and HCO_3^- secretion, reabsorption, and conservation, and ammonia synthesis for excretion in the urine. H^+ secretion is regulated by the amount of carbon dioxide in extracellular fluid: the greater the concentration of carbon dioxide, the greater the amount of H^+ secretion, resulting in an acidic urine. When H^+ is excreted, bicarbonate is generated by the kidneys, helping to maintain the 1:20 balance of acids and bases. When extracellular fluid is alkalotic, the kidneys conserve H^+ and eliminate sodium bicarbonate, resulting in alkalotic urine. Although the kidneys' response to an abnormal pH is slow (several hours to days), healthy kidneys usually are able to adjust the imbalance

Table 12-1   Normal arterial and venous blood gas values

	Arterial Values		Venous Values
	Perfect	Range	
pH	7.40	7.35-7.45	pH 7.32-7.38
$Paco_2$	40 mm Hg	35-45 mm Hg	Pco_2 42-50 mm Hg
Pao_2	95 mm Hg	80-100 mm Hg	Po_2 40 mm Hg
Saturation	95%-99%		Saturation 75%
Base excess	+ or −2		
*Serum HCO_3^-	24 mEq/L	22-26 mEq/L	HCO_3^- 23-27 mEq/L

*Although serum bicarbonate is a buffer, it is usually reported as CO_2 content or total CO_2 and not as serum HCO_3^-. The serum HCO_3^- concentration usually is obtained separately from ABG analysis and is critical in the determination of acid-base status. Values should be obtained with the initial ABG assessment and daily thereafter.

$Paco_2$ = carbon dioxide tension of arterial blood; PaO_2 = oxygen tension of arterial blood; HCO_3^- = bicarbonate ion; Pco_2 = carbon dioxide partial pressure; PO_2 = partial pressure of oxygen.

Table 12-2   ABG comparisons of acid-base disorders

		Alkalosis			Acidosis		
		$Paco_2$	pH	HCO_3^-	$Paco_2$	pH	HCO_3^-
Simple	Respiratory	25	*7.60	24	50	*7.15	25
	Metabolic	44	7.54	36	38	7.20	15
Compensated	Respiratory	25	7.54	21	66	7.37	34
	Metabolic	50	7.42	31	23	7.28	9
Mixed Disorder		40	7.56	38	50	7.20	20

*Note the greater changes in pH with acute respiratory disorders owing to delayed renal compensation.

Table 12-3 Quick assessment guide to acid-base imbalances

Acid-Base Imbalance	pH	Pa_{CO_2}	HCO_3^-
Acute respiratory acidosis	Decreased	Increased	No change
Chronic respiratory acidosis (compensated)	Decreased	Increased	Increased*
Acute respiratory alkalosis	Increased	Decreased	No change (a decrease will occur if condition has been present for hours, providing that renal function is adequate)
Chronic respiratory alkalosis	Increased	Decreased	Decreased*
Acute metabolic acidosis	Decreased	Decreased*	Decreased
Chronic metabolic acidosis	Decreased	Decreased* (not as much as acute type)	Decreased

*Compensatory response.

Clinical Signs and Symptoms	Common Causes
Tachycardia, tachypnea, diaphoresis, headache, restlessness leading to lethargy and coma, cyanosis, dysrhythmias, hypotension.	Acute respiratory failure, cardiopulmonary disease, drug overdose, chest wall trauma, asphyxiation, CNS trauma/lesions, impaired muscles of respiration.
Dyspnea and tachypnea, with increase in CO_2 retention that exceeds compensatory ability; progression to lethargy, confusion, and coma.	COPD, extreme obesity (Pickwickian syndrome), superimposed infection on COPD.
Paresthesias, especially of the fingers; dizziness.	Hyperventilation, salicylate poisoning, hypoxia (e.g., with pneumonia, pulmonary edema, pulmonary thromboembolism), gram negative sepsis, CNS lesion, decreased lung compliance, inappropriate mechanical ventilation.
No symptoms	Hepatic failure; CNS lesion.
Tachypnea leading to Kussmaul respirations, hypotension, cold and clammy skin, coma, and dysrhythmias.	Shock, cardiopulmonary arrest (secondary to lactic acid production), ketoacidosis (e.g., diabetes, starvation, alcohol abuse), acute renal failure, ingestion of acids (e.g., salicylates), diarrhea.
Fatigue, anorexia, malaise. Symptoms may be related to chronic disease process as well as acidosis.	Chronic renal failure.

COPD = chronic obstructive pulmonary disease; CNS = central nervous system; Cl^- = chloride ion; Na^+ = sodium ion; K^+ = potassium ion

Table continued on p. 146.

Table 12-3 *(continued)*

Acid-Base Imbalance	pH	Paco$_2$	HCO$_3^-$
Acute metabolic alkalosis	Increased	Increased* (can be as great as 60)	Increased
Chronic metabolic alkalosis	Increased	Increased*	Increased

*Compensatory response.

to normal because of their ability to excrete large quantities of excess bicarbonate and H$^+$ from the body.

Blood Gas Values

Blood gas analysis usually is based on arterial sampling. Venous values are given as a reference (see Table 12-1, p. 142).

Arterial Blood Gas (ABG) Analysis

ABG measurement is the best means of evaluating acid-base balance.

1. **pH:** Measures H$^+$ concentration to reflect acid-base status of the blood. Values reflect whether arterial pH is normal (7.40), acidic (<7.40), or alkalotic (>7.40). Because of the ability of compensatory mechanisms to "normalize" the pH, a near-normal value does not exclude the possibility of an acid-base disturbance.

Clinical Signs and Symptoms	Common Causes
Muscular weakness and hyporeflexia (due to severe hypokalemia), dysrhythmias, apathy, confusion, and stupor.	Volume depletion (Cl^- depletion) as a result of vomiting, gastric drainage, diuretic use, post-hypercapnia. Hyperadrenocorticism (e.g., Cushing's syndrome), aldosteronism, severe potassium depletion, excessive alkali intake.
Usually asymptomatic.	Upper GI losses through continuous drainage; correction of hypercapnia if Na^+ and K^+ depletion remains uncorrected.

COPD = chronic obstructive pulmonary disease; CNS = central nervous system; Cl^- = chloride ion; Na^+ = sodium ion; K^+ = potassium ion.

2. **$Paco_2$:** Partial pressure of carbon dioxide in the arteries. It is the respiratory component of acid-base regulation and is adjusted by changes in the rate and depth of pulmonary ventilation. Hypercapnia ($Paco_2 > 45$ mm Hg) indicates alveolar hypoventilation and respiratory acidosis. Hyperventilation results in a $Paco_2 < 35$ mm Hg and respiratory alkalosis. Respiratory compensation occurs rapidly in metabolic acid-base disturbances. If any abnormality in $Paco_2$ exists, it is important to analyze pH and HCO_3^- parameters to determine if the alteration in $Paco_2$ is the result of a primary respiratory disturbance or a compensatory response to a metabolic acid-base abnormality.

3. **Pao_2:** Partial pressure of oxygen in the arteries. It has no primary role in acid-base regulation if it is within normal limits. The presence of hypoxemia with a $Pao_2 < 60$ mm Hg can lead to anaerobic metabolism, resulting in lactic acid production and metabolic acidosis. There is a normal decline in Pao_2 in the aged. Hypoxemia also may cause hyperventilation resulting in respiratory alkalosis.

Table 12-4 Acid-base rules: general guidelines

Disturbance	Change in pH	Compensatory Response	Results of Compensation
Respiratory acidosis			
Acute	pH $\downarrow$ 0.08 for every 10 mm Hg $\uparrow$ in $Paco_2$	Immediate release of tissue buffers (i.e., HCO_3^-)	1.0 mEq/L $\uparrow$ in HCO_3^- from patient's baseline for every 10 mm Hg $\uparrow$ in $Paco_2$
Chronic	Depends on renal compensation; often near normal	$\uparrow$ Renal reabsorption of HCO_3^-; clinically evident after 8 hr; maximal effect 3-5 days	3.5 mEq/L $\uparrow$ in HCO_3^-, for every 10 mm Hg $\uparrow$ in $Paco_2$
Respiratory alkalosis			
Acute	pH $\uparrow$ 0.08 for every 10 mm Hg $\downarrow$ in $Paco_2$	Immediate release of tissue buffers	2.0 mEq/L $\downarrow$ in HCO_3^- from patient's baseline for every 10 mm Hg $\downarrow$ in $Paco_2$
Chronic	pH can be returned to normal if renal function is adequate	$\downarrow$ Renal reabsorption of HCO_3^-	Maximal renal compensation causes HCO_3^-; to $\downarrow$ 5 mEq/L for every 10 mm Hg $\downarrow$ in $Paco_2$. Maximal effect can take 7-9 days and may *normalize* pH

Metabolic acidosis			
Acute	pH ↓ 0.15 for every 10 mEq/L ↓ in HCO_3^-	Hyperventilation occurs immediately	1.2 mm Hg ↓ in $Paco_2$ for every 1 mEq/L ↓ in HCO_3^-
Chronic	pH same as it would be if no respiratory compensation were present	Hyperventilation	The effects of hyperventilation last only a few days because the ↓ in $Paco_2$ causes a further ↓ in renal reabsorption of HCO_3^-
Metabolic alkalosis			
Acute	pH ↑ 0.15 for every 10 mEq/L ↑ in HCO_3^-	Hypoventilation occurs immediately	0.7 mm Hg ↑ in $Paco_2$ for every 1 mEq/L ↑ in HCO_3^-
Chronic	pH same as it would be if respiratory compensation were present	Hypoventilation	The effects of hypoventilation last for only a few days because the ↑ in $Paco_2$ causes ↑ renal excretion of H^+ and ↑ serum HCO_3^-.

4. **Saturation:** Measures the degree to which hemoglobin is saturated by oxygen. It can be affected by changes in temperature, pH, and $Paco_2$. When the Pao_2 falls below 60 mm Hg, there is a large drop in saturation.

5. **Base excess or deficit:** Indicates, in general terms, the amount of blood buffer (hemoglobin and plasma bicarbonate) present. Abnormally high values reflect alkalosis; low values reflect acidosis. Normal value is $\pm$ 2.

6. **HCO_3^-:** Serum bicarbonate is the major renal component of acid-base regulation. It is excreted or regenerated by the kidneys to maintain a normal acid-base environment. Decreased bicarbonate levels (<22 mEq/L) are indicative of metabolic acidosis (seen infrequently as a compensatory mechanism for respiratory alkalosis); elevated bicarbonate levels (>26 mEq/L) reflect metabolic alkalosis—either as a primary metabolic disorder or as a compensatory alteration in response to respiratory acidosis.

Step-by-Step Guide to ABG Analysis

A systematic step-by-step analysis critical to the accurate interpretation of ABG values. For further information, see Tables 12-2, 12-3, and 12-4 (pp. 143, 144, and 148).

1. **Step one:** Determine if pH is normal. If it deviates from 7.40, note how much it deviates and in which direction. For example, pH >7.40 indicates alkalosis; pH <7.40 indicates acidosis. Is the pH in the normal range of 7.35 to 7.45 or is it in the critical range of >7.55 or <7.20?

2. **Step two:** Check the $Paco_2$. If it deviates from 40 mm Hg, how much does it deviate and in which direction? Does the change in $Paco_2$ correspond to the direction of the change in pH? The pH and $Paco_2$ should move in opposite directions. For example, as the $Paco_2$ increases, the pH should decrease (acidosis); and as the $Paco_2$ decreases, the pH should increase (alkalosis).

3. **Step three:** Determine the HCO_3^- value (may be referred to as total CO_2 content, serum CO_2, or serum HCO_3^-). If it deviates from 24 mEq/L, note the degree and direction of deviation. Does the change in HCO_3^- correspond to the change in pH? The HCO_3^- and pH should move in the same direction. For example, if the HCO_3^- decreases, the

pH should decrease (acidosis); and as the HCO_3^- increases, the pH should increase (alkalosis).

4. **Step four:** If both the $Paco_2$ and HCO_3^-; are abnormal, which value corresponds more closely to the pH value? For example, if the pH reflects acidosis, which value also reflects acidosis (an increased $Paco_2$ or a decreased HCO_3^-)? The value that more closely corresponds to the pH and deviates more from normal points to the primary disturbance responsible for the alteration in pH. A mixed metabolic-respiratory disturbance or compensatory elements may be present when both HCO_3^- and $Paco_2$ are abnormal.

5. **Step five:** Check Pao_2 and oxygen saturation to determine whether they are decreased, normal, or increased. Decreased Pao_2 and O_2 saturation can lead to lactic acidosis and may signal the need for increased concentrations of oxygen. Conversely, high Pao_2 may be indicative of the need to decrease delivered concentrations of oxygen.

Arterial-Venous Difference

The difference between arterial oxygen content and venous oxygen content reflects the tissue extraction of oxygen. The normal value for arterial oxygen content is 18 ml/100 ml blood, whereas the normal value for venous blood or pulmonary artery oxygen content is 14 ml/100 ml blood. The difference between these two values increases when ventricular performance is impaired, for example, right ventricular failure associated with congestive heart failure.

Respiratory Acidosis

13

Acute Respiratory Acidosis

Respiratory acidosis occurs secondary to alveolar hypoventilation and results in a carbon dioxide tension of arterial blood (Pa_{CO_2}) >40 mm Hg (hypercapnia) and a pH <7.40. Pa_{CO_2} derangements are direct reflections of the degree of ventilatory dysfunction. Normally, carbon dioxide (CO_2) excretion equals CO_2 production. When there is an excess amount of CO_2, the lungs are failing to eliminate the necessary amount to maintain the Pa_{CO_2} at 40 mm Hg. The degree to which the increased Pa_{CO_2} alters the pH depends on both the rapidity of onset and the body's ability to compensate through the blood buffer and renal systems. Although the blood buffer system acts immediately, it usually is not sufficient to maintain a normal pH in the presence of an elevated Pa_{CO_2}. There is a delay (hours to days) before the effects of renal compensation can be noted, so acute respiratory acidosis can have a profound impact on pH.

Assessment

1. **Signs and symptoms:** Dyspnea; asterixis; restlessness leading to lethargy, confusion, and coma.
2. **Physical assessment:** Increased heart and respiratory rates, diaphoresis, and cyanosis. Severe hypercapnia may cause cerebral vasodilatation, resulting in increased intracranial pressure (ICP) with papilledema. Another finding may be dilated conjunctival and facial blood vessels.
3. **Monitoring parameters:** Presence of ventricular dysrhythmias; increased ICP.
4. **History and risk factors:** See also the box opposite.
   - *Acute respiratory disease:* Acute respiratory failure from a number of causes, including pneumonia, adult respiratory distress syndrome (ARDS).

- *Overdose of drugs:* Oversedation with drugs that cause respiratory center depression.
- *Chest wall trauma:* Flail chest, pneumothorax.
- *Central nervous-system trauma/lesions:* Can lead to depression of respiratory center.
- *Asphyxiation:* Mechanical obstruction; anaphylaxis.
- *Impaired respiratory muscles:* Can occur with hyperkalemia, polio, Guillain-Barré syndrome.
- *Iatrogenic:* Inappropriate mechanical ventilation (increased dead space, insufficient rate or volume); high fraction of inspired oxygen (FIo_2) in the presence of chronic CO_2 retention.

Potential Causes of Acute Respiratory Acidosis

Pulmonary/Thoracic Disorders

Severe pneumonia
ARDS
Flail chest
Pneumothorax
Hemothorax
Smoke inhalation

Airway Obstruction

Aspiration
Laryngospasm (anaphylaxis, severe hypocalcemia)
Severe bronchospasm
Severe, prolonged acute asthma attack

CNS Depression

Sedative overdose
Anesthesia
Cerebral trauma
Cerebral infarct

Metabolic Causes

High-carbohydrate diet

Neuromuscular Abnormalities

Guillain-Barré syndrome
Hypokalemia
High-cervical cordotomy
Drugs (e.g., curare)
Toxins

Systemic Causes

Cardiac arrest
Massive pulmonary embolus
Severe pulmonary edema

Mechanical Ventilation

Fixed minute ventilation with increased CO_2 production
Inappropriate dead space
Equipment failure

Diagnostic Tests

1. **Arterial blood gas (ABG) analysis:** Aids in diagnosis and determination of severity of respiratory acidosis. $Paco_2$ will be >40 mm Hg and pH will be <7.40. All individuals with elevated $Paco_2$ will have some degree of hypoxemia while breathing room air.
2. **Serum bicarbonate (also referred to as serum CO_2):** Reflects metabolic and base balance. Initially, bicarbonate ion (HCO_3^-) values will be normal (22-26 mEq/L) unless a mixed disorder is present.
3. **Serum electrolytes:** Usually not altered, depending on etiology of respiratory acidosis.
4. **Chest x-ray:** Determines presence of underlying respiratory disease.
5. **Drug screen:** Determines presence and quantity of drug if patient is suspected of taking an overdose.

Collaborative Management

1. **Restoration of normal acid-base balance:** Accomplished by supporting respiratory function. If $Paco_2$ is >50-60 mm Hg and clinical signs such as cyanosis and lethargy are present, the patient usually requires intubation and mechanical ventilation. Generally, use of bicarbonate is avoided because of the risk of alkalosis when the respiratory disturbance has been corrected. Although a life-threatening pH must be corrected promptly to an acceptable level, a normal pH is not the immediate goal.
2. **Treatment of underlying disorder.**

ndx: Nursing Diagnoses and Interventions

Impaired gas exchange related to alveolar hypoventilation secondary to underlying disease process
Desired outcome: Patient has adequate gas exchange as evidenced by oxygen tension of arterial blood (Pao_2) ≥ 60 mm Hg, $Paco_2$ ≤ 45 mm Hg, pH 7.35-7.45, RR 12-20 breaths/min with a normal pattern and depth (eupnea), and absence of adventitious breath sounds.

1. Monitor serial ABG results to detect continued presence of hypercapnia or hypoxemia. Report significant findings (i.e., variances of 10-20 mm Hg in $Paco_2$ or Pao_2.

2. Assess and document character of respiratory effort: rate, depth, rhythm, and use of accessory muscles of respiration.

3. Assess patient for signs and symptoms of respiratory distress: restlessness, anxiety, confusion, and tachypnea (respiratory rate >20 breaths/min).

4. Position patient for comfort and to ensure optimal gas exchange. Usually, semi-Fowler's position allows for adequate expansion of the chest wall, but the specific pathologic process must be considered when positioning patients.

   - For unilateral lung disease in the patient who is ventilated mechanically, a side-lying (lateral decubitus) position may increase perfusion in the dependent (healthy) lung and increase ventilation to the upper (diseased) lung.

   - For patients with ARDS requiring mechanical ventilation, the prone position may improve gas exchange by decreasing the edema and increasing the ventilation to the dependent lung area (Langer, 1988). Hypoventilation can occur in dependent areas with mechanical ventilation, resulting in atelectasis. Not all patients with ARDS will benefit from the prone position and a brief trial (30 minutes) in this position is recommended to identify patients who can benefit from it. Improved ventilatory status will be noted by improvement in breath sounds and ABG values (increased Pao_2 on same oxygen concentration and ventilator settings).

Sensory-perceptual alterations related to disturbance in acid-base regulation

Desired outcome: Patient verbalizes orientation to person, place, and time and does not exhibit evidence of injury caused by altered sensorium.

1. Monitor ABG and serum CO_2 results. Notify MD regarding abnormal values and significant changes (that is, variances of 10-20 mm Hg in Pao_2 and $Paco_2$). At frequent intervals assess and document the patient's level of consciousness (LOC) and orientation to person, place, and time.

2. Use reality therapy, such as familiar photos, a calendar, and a clock with a face that is large enough for patient to

see. Keep these items at the bedside and within the patient's visual field.

3. Keep the bed in its lowest position, with all siderails up and the wheels locked.

4. If patient is allowed out of bed, remind patient to ask for assistance before getting up.

5. Offer confused patients the opportunity to toilet at frequent intervals. Many falls result from disoriented or unsteady patients' attempts to toilet.

6. Use a night light to minimize confusion in an unfamiliar and unlit environment.

7. If patient's confusion persists despite reorientation, increase the frequency of observations, with concomitant reorientation and documentation. Alert MD to continued or increasing confusion.

8. Reassure patient's significant others that patient's confusion will abate with treatment.

9. If patient remains at risk for injury, obtain a prescription for a protective restraining device per agency policy.

   - Document need for restraining device based on patient's behavior upon initiation and every 8 hours thereafter.
   - Choose the least restrictive device that will protect patient. Add additional device(s) as needed, based on documented patient behaviors.
   - Document type of device used. A protective vest is applied to the upper torso with the crisscross or "V" in the front. Soft limb protectors are applied to the upper extremities (may be applied to upper and lower extremities in some cases).
   - Monitor patient every 15-30 minutes while restraints are in use, documenting mental status and response to protective device(s).
   - Document frequency (at least every 2 hours) of device removal, repositioning of patient, and reapplication of the device.

Altered oral mucous membrane related to abnormal breathing pattern
Desired outcome: Patient's oral mucosa, lips, and tongue are intact with adequate moisture.

1. Assess patient's oral mucous membrane, lips, and tongue

every 2 hours, noting presence of dryness, exudate, swelling, blisters, and ulcers.

2. If patient is alert and able to take fluids orally, offer frequent sips of water or ice chips to alleviate dryness.

3. Perform mouth care every 2-4 hours, using a soft-bristled toothbrush to cleanse the teeth and a moistened cloth or toothette (small sponge on a stick) to moisten crusty areas or exudate on the tongue and oral mucosa. If patient is intubated, suction the mouth to remove fluid and debris.

4. If indicated, use an artificial saliva preparation to assist in keeping mucous membrane moist. Avoid use of lemon and glycerine swabs, which can contribute to dryness.

Sleep pattern disturbance related to frequent treatments and procedures
Desired outcome: Patient sleeps undisturbed for at least 90 minutes at a time and relates a feeling of well being.

1. Gather information about patient's normal sleep habits: bedtime rituals; usual position; hours of sleep required; number of pillows used; sensitivity to light, noise, and touch. Based on data gathered, attempt to incorporate patient's needs into his or her care plan.

2. Cluster activities and procedure to minimize need for interrupting patient's sleep. Even brief (30-second) interruptions of sleep can result in feelings of fatigue.

3. Attempt to administer unpleasant or uncomfortable procedures or treatments at least one hour before bedtime to allow time for relaxation before patient attempts to go to sleep.

4. Offer backrubs, repositioning, and relaxation techniques (quiet music, instructions for imagery) at bedtime.

5. If patient requires a daytime nap owing to fatigue, provide opportunities to sleep between 1 PM and 3 PM. Sleep attained at this time is most restful and least likely to disrupt night-time sleep. Discourage napping after 7 PM, as it may prevent patient from falling asleep and maintaining a normal sleep cycle.

Ineffective family coping related to stress reaction secondary to catastrophic illness of family member
Desired outcome: Family members exhibit effective coping

mechanisms, seek support from others, and discuss concerns among the family unit.

1. Establish an open line of communication with the family, providing an atmosphere in which family members can ask questions, ventilate feelings, and discuss concerns among other family members.
2. Assess family members' knowledge about patient's therapies and treatments. Provide information, as needed, and reinforce information family has received from other health care members.
3. Provide opportunities and areas for family members to talk privately as well as share concerns with health care members.
4. Determine effective coping strategies that have been used by the family in other stressful situations. Support and encourage family to continue use of healthy, effective coping strategies.
5. Enable family members to spend time alone with patient for short, frequent intervals.
6. Encourage family members to pursue diversional activities outside the hospital to help alleviate stress of the immediate situation. Families often feel the need for "permission" from health care members to leave the waiting room or hospital.
7. Offer realistic hope.

Chronic Respiratory Acidosis (Compensated)

This disorder occurs in pulmonary diseases (e.g., chronic emphysema and bronchitis) in which effective alveolar ventilation is decreased and a ventilation-perfusion mismatch is present. Chronic hypercapnia also can occur with obesity. In patients with a chronic lung disease, a nearly normal pH can be seen if renal function is normal, even if the $Paco_2$ is as high as 60 mm Hg. Chronic compensatory metabolic alkalosis (serum HCO_3^- >26 mEq/L) occurs and maintains an acceptable acid-base environment, which results in compensated respiratory acidosis and a normal or near normal pH. Patients with chronic lung disease can experience acute rises in $Paco_2$ secondary to superimposed disease states such as pneumonia. If the chronic compensatory mechanisms in place (e.g., elevated HCO_3^-) are inadequate to meet the sudden increase in $Paco_2$, decompensation may occur with a resultant decrease in pH.

Assessment

1. **Signs and symptoms:** If the $Paco_2$ does not exceed the body's ability to compensate, no specific findings will be noted. If $Paco_2$ rises rapidly, the following may occur: dull headache, weakness, dyspnea, asterixis, agitation, and insomnia progressing to somnolence and coma.
2. **Physical assessment:** Tachypnea, cyanosis. Severe hypercapnia ($Paco_2$ >70 mm Hg) may cause cerebral vasodilation resulting in increased ICP, papilledema, and dilated conjunctival and facial blood vessels. Depending on underlying pathophysiology, edema may be present secondary to right ventricular failure.
3. **History and risk factors** (See also accompanying box).
   - *Chronic obstructive pulmonary disease (COPD):* Predominantly emphysema and bronchitis.
   - *Extreme obesity:* Pickwickian syndrome.

Potential Causes of Chronic Respiratory Acidosis

Obstructive Diseases

Emphysema
Chronic bronchitis
Cystic fibrosis
Obstructive sleep apnea

Restriction of Ventilation

Kyphoscoliosis
Hydrothorax
Fibrothorax
Severe chronic
   pneumonitis
Obesity-hypoventilation
   (Pickwickian) syndrome

Neuromuscular Abnormalities

Poliomyelitis
Muscular dystrophy
Multiple sclerosis
Amyotrophic lateral sclerosis (ALS)
Diaphragmatic paralysis

Depression of the Respiratory Center

Brain tumor
Bulbar poliomyelitis
Chronic sedative overdose
Obesity-hypoventilation
   (Pickwickian) syndrome

- *Development of superimposed acute respiratory infection in a patient with COPD.*
- *Exposure to pulmonary toxins:* Occupational risk; pollution.

Diagnostic Tests

1. **ABG values:** Provide data necessary for determining the diagnosis and severity of respiratory acidosis. Although the $Paco_2$ will be elevated, the pH will be on the acidic (low) side of normal owing to renal compensation, except in patients who are experiencing acute pulmonary infection. If the $Paco_2$ has increased abruptly from baseline value, a pH lower than normal may be seen.
2. **Serum bicarbonate:** HCO_3^- (serum CO_2) is especially helpful in determining the level of metabolic compensation that has occurred (i.e., increased HCO_3^- with a near normal pH if fully compensated). This information is particularly useful in identifying "mixed" acid-base disturbances (see Chapter 17) because the HCO_3^- is expected to be elevated in chronic respiratory acidosis. If the HCO_3^- is normal or low, this could be diagnostic of a pathologic process concurrent with the first.
3. **Chest x-ray:** Determines extent of underlying pulmonary disease and identifies further pathologic changes that may be responsible for acute exacerbation, (e.g., pneumonia).
4. **Electrocardiogram (ECG):** Identifies cardiac involvement from COPD. For example, right-sided heart failure is a complication of chronic bronchitis.
5. **Sputum culture:** Determines presence of pathogens causing an acute exacerbation of a chronic pulmonary disease (e.g., pneumonia) present in a patient with COPD.

Collaborative Management

1. **Oxygen therapy:** Used cautiously (i.e., not greater than 3 L/min) in patients with chronic CO_2 retention for whom hypoxia, rather than hypercapnia, stimulates ventilation. Patient may require intubation and mechanical ventilation for stupor and coma precipitated by oxygen if the drive to breathe is eliminated by high concentrations of oxygen.
2. **Pharmacotherapy:** Bronchodilators and antibiotics, as in-

dicated. Narcotics and sedatives can depress the respiratory center and are avoided unless patient is intubated and mechanically ventilated.

3. **IV fluids:** Maintain adequate hydration for mobilizing pulmonary secretions.
4. **Chest physiotherapy:** Aids in expectoration of sputum; includes postural drainage if hypersecretions are present. Assess patient closely during this procedure because it may be poorly tolerated, especially the postural drainage component.

Nursing Diagnoses and Interventions

Impaired gas exchange related to trapping of CO_2 secondary to pulmonary tissue destruction (appropriate for the patient with COPD)

Desired outcome: ABG values reflect a $Paco_2$ and pH within acceptable range, based on patient's underlying pulmonary disease.

1. Monitor serial ABG results to assess patient's response to therapy. Report significant findings to MD: an increasing $Paco_2$ and a decreasing pH.
2. Assess and document patient's respiratory status: respiratory rate and rhythm, exertional effort, and breath sounds. Compare pretreatment findings to posttreatment (e.g., oxygen therapy, physiotherapy, or medications) findings for evidence of improvement.
3. Assess and document patient's LOC. If $Paco_2$ increases, be alert to subtle, progressive changes in mental status. A common progression is agitation→ insomnia→ somnolence→ coma. To avoid a comatose state secondary to rising CO_2 levels, always evaluate the "arousability" of a patient with elevated $Paco_2$ who appears to be sleeping. Notify MD if patient is difficult to arouse.
4. Ensure appropriate delivery of prescribed oxygen therapy. Assess patient's respiratory status after every change in FIo_2. Patients with chronic CO_2 retention may be very sensitive to increases in FIo_2, resulting in depressed ventilatory drive. If patient requires mechanical ventilation, be aware of the importance of maintaining the compensated acid base environment. If the $Paco_2$ were rapidly decreased by a high respiratory rate per mechanical ventilation, a severe metabolic alkalosis could develop. The sudden onset of metabolic alka-

losis may lead to hypocalcemia, which can result in tetany (see "Hypocalcemia," p. 109).

5. Assess for presence of bowel sounds and monitor for gastric distention, which can impede movement of the diaphragm and restrict ventilatory effort further.

6. If patient is not intubated, encourage use of pursed-lip breathing (inhalation through nose, with slow exhalation through pursed lips), which helps airways to remain open and allows for better air excursion. Optimally, this technique will diminish air entrapment in the lungs and make respiratory effort more efficient.

Ineffective airway clearance related to viscous secretions and fatigue

Desired outcome: Auscultation of patient's airway reveals the absence of adventitious breath sounds.

1. Be alert to increased fatigue or lethargy as a potential sign of increasing $Paco_2$.

2. If patient is unable to raise secretions independently, perform suctioning as often as its need is determined by assessment findings.

3. If prescribed, administer chest physiotherapy. (Chest physiotherapy may be contraindicated in some patients with chronic CO_2 retention.) Evaluate effectiveness of therapy by assessing breath sounds, ABG results, and patency of airway both before and after treatment.

4. Ensure adequate fluid intake to compensate for increased insensible losses owing to increased respiratory rate, febrile state, and diaphoresis. Adequate hydration will make secretions less viscous and easier to mobilize.

5. Encourage nonintubated patient to continue with pursed-lip breathing (inhalation through nose, with slow exhalation through pursed lips), which will increase efficiency and effectiveness of respiratory effort.

For other nursing diagnoses and interventions, see "Acute Respiratory Acidosis" for the following: **Altered oral mucous membrane** related to abnormal breathing pattern (see p. 156), and **Sleep pattern disturbance** related to frequent treatments and procedures (see p. 157).

Respiratory Alkalosis 14

Acute Respiratory Alkalosis

Respiratory alkalosis occurs as a result of an increase in the rate of alveolar ventilation (alveolar hyperventilation). It is defined by carbon dioxide tension of arterial blood ($Paco_2$) <40 mm Hg (hypocapnia) and a pH >7.40. Acute alveolar hyperventilation most frequently is the result of anxiety and is commonly referred to as "hyperventilation syndrome." In addition, numerous physiologic disorders (see "History and risk factors," below) can cause acute hypocapnia, which results in increased pH. The rise in pH is modified to a small degree by intracellular buffering. To compensate for increased carbon dioxide (CO_2) loss and the resultant base excess, hydrogen ions are released from tissue buffers, which in turn lower plasma bicarbonate concentration. The kidney's response to respiratory alkalosis is slow (several hours to days), and thus acute respiratory alkalosis usually is resolved before renal compensation can occur.

Assessment

1. **Signs and symptoms:** Lightheadedness, anxiety, paresthesias, circumoral numbness. In extreme alkalosis, confusion, tetany, syncope, and seizures may occur.
2. **Physical assessment:** Increased rate and depth of respirations.
3. **Electrocardiogram (ECG) findings:** Cardiac dysrhythmias.
4. **History and risk factors** (see also the box on p. 164):
   - *Anxiety:* Patient is often unaware of hyperventilation.
   - *Acute hypoxia:* Pulmonary disorders (e.g., pneumonia, pulmonary edema, and pulmonary thromboembolism)

Potential Causes of Acute Respiratory Alkalosis

Hypoxemia	**Central (Direct) Stimulation of the Respiratory Center**
Pneumonia	
High altitude (>6500 feet)	
Hypotension	Anxiety
Severe anemia	Fever
Congestive heart failure	Pain
	Drugs (salicylates)
Pulmonary Disorders	Voluntary or mechanical hyperventilation
Pulmonary emboli	Intracerebral trauma
Inhalation of irritants	Gram-negative septicemia
Interstitial fibrosis	Acute cerebral vascular
Pneumonia	accident
Pulmonary edema	
Asthma	

cause hypoxia, which stimulates the ventilatory effort in the initial stages of the disease process.

- *Hypermetabolic states:* Fever; sepsis, especially gram-negative induced septicemia.
- *Salicylate intoxication*
- *Excessive mechanical ventilation.*
- *Central Nervous System (CNS) trauma:* May result in damage to respiratory center.

Diagnostic Tests

1. **Arterial blood gas (ABG) values:** $Paco_2$ <40 mm Hg and pH >7.40 will be present. A decreased oxygen tension of arterial blood (Pao_2), along with the clinical picture (e.g., pneumonia, pulmonary edema, pulmonary embolism, and adult respiratory distress syndrome), may help diagnose the etiology of the respiratory alkalosis.
2. **Serum electrolytes:** Determine presence of metabolic acid-base disorders.
3. **Serum phosphate:** May fall to less than 0.5 mg/dl (normal is 3.0-4.5 mg/dl) owing to the alkalosis, which causes increased uptake of phosphate by the cells.

4. **ECG:** Detects cardiac dysrhythmias, which may be present with alkalosis.

Collaborative Management

1. **Treatment of underlying disorder.**
2. **Reassurance:** If anxiety is the cause of decreased $Paco_2$. If symptoms are severe, it may be necessary for patient to re-breathe CO_2 through an oxygen mask with an attached CO_2 reservoir. If such a device is not readily available, breathing into a paper bag will produce the same effect.
3. **Oxygen therapy:** If hypoxia is the causative factor.
4. **Adjustments to mechanical ventilators:** Settings are checked and adjustments made to ventilatory parameters in response to ABG results that signal hypocapnia. Respiratory rate or volume is decreased and dead space is added, if necessary.
5. **Pharmacotherapy:** Sedatives and tranquilizers may be given for anxiety-induced respiratory alkalosis.

Nursing Diagnoses and Interventions

ndx:

Ineffective breathing pattern related to hyperventilation secondary to anxiety
Desired outcome: Patient's breathing pattern is effective as evidenced by a $Paco_2$ ≥35 mm Hg and a pH ≤7.45.

1. To help alleviate anxiety, reassure patient that a staff member will remain with him or her.
2. Encourage patient to breathe slowly. Pace patient's breathing by having him or her mimic your own breathing pattern.
3. Monitor patient's cardiac rhythm, notifying MD if dysrhythmias occur. With acute respiratory alkalosis, even a modest alkalosis can precipitate dysrhythmias in a patient with a pre-existing heart disease who is also taking cardiotropic drugs.
4. Administer sedatives or tranquilizers as prescribed.
5. Have patient rebreathe into a paper bag or into an oxygen mask with an attached CO_2 reservoir, if prescribed.
6. Ensure that patient rests undisturbed after his or her

breathing pattern has stabilized. Hyperventilation can result in fatigue.

Note: Hyperventilation may lead to hypocalcemic tetany despite a normal or near normal calcium level due to increased binding of calcium (see Chapter 9).

Chronic Respiratory Alkalosis

This is a state of chronic hypocapnia, which stimulates the renal compensatory response and results in a decrease in plasma bicarbonate. Maximal renal compensatory response requires several days to occur.

Assessment

1. **Signs and symptoms:** Individuals with chronic respiratory alkalosis usually are asymptomatic.
2. **Physical assessment:** Increased respiratory rate and depth.
3. **History and risk factors:**
   - *Cerebral disease:* Tumor, encephalitis.
   - *Chronic hepatic insufficiency.*
   - *Pregnancy.*
   - *Chronic hypoxia:* Adaptation to high altitude; cyanotic heart disease; lung disease resulting in decreased compliance (e.g., fibrosis).

Diagnostic Tests

1. **ABG values:** $Paco_2$ will be <35 mm Hg, with a nearly normal pH; Pao_2 may be decreased if hypoxia is the causative factor.
2. **Serum electrolytes:** Probably will be normal, with the exception of plasma bicarbonate (HCO_3^-), which will decrease as renal compensation occurs. Maximal renal compensation takes 7–9 days with normalization of pH.
3. **Phosphate levels:** Hypophosphatemia (as low as 0.5 mg/dl) may be seen with intense hyperventilation. Alkalosis causes increased uptake of phosphate by the cells.

Collaborative Management

1. **Treatment of underlying cause.**
2. **Oxygen therapy:** If hypoxia is present and identified as causative factor in respiratory alkalosis.

Nursing Diagnoses and Interventions

Nursing diagnoses and interventions are specific to the pathophysiologic process.

Metabolic Acidosis

15

Acute Metabolic Acidosis

Metabolic acidosis is caused by a primary decrease in plasma bicarbonate, as reflected by a serum bicarbonate of <22 mEq/L with a pH <7.40. The decrease in serum bicarbonate is caused by one of the following mechanisms: (1) increase in the concentration of hydrogen ions in the form of nonvolatile acids (e.g., ketoacidosis associated with diabetes and alcoholism; lactic acidosis); (2) loss of alkali (e.g., severe diarrhea, intestinal malabsorption); (3) decreased acid excretion by the kidneys (e.g., acute and chronic renal failure). The decrease in pH stimulates respirations. The body's attempts to compensate occur rapidly, as manifested by lowering of the carbon dioxide tension of arterial blood ($Paco_2$), which may be reduced by as much as 10-15 mm Hg. The most important mechanism for ridding the body of excess hydrogen ions (H^+) is the increase in acid excretion by the kidneys. However, nonvolatile acids may accumulate more rapidly than they can be neutralized by the body's buffers, compensated for by the respiratory system, or excreted by the kidneys.

Assessment

1. **Signs and symptoms:** Findings vary, depending on underlying disease states and severity of acid-base disturbance. There may be changes in level of consciousness that range from fatigue and confusion to stupor and coma.
2. **Physical assessment:** Decreased blood pressure, tachypnea leading to alveolar hyperventilation (Kussmaul's respirations), cold and clammy skin, presence of dysrhythmias, and shock state.
3. **History and risk factors** (see accompanying box):
   - *Renal disease:* Acute renal failure.

Potential Causes of Metabolic Acidosis

Loss of HCO_3^-	Excess Acid Production/Ingestion	Inability of the Kidneys to Excrete Acid (H^+) Load
Gastrointestinal	**Ketoacidosis**	**Renal insufficiency; acute or chronic renal failure**
1. Diarrhea	1. Diabetic	
2. Biliary and pancreatic drainage	2. Alcohol induced	
3. Urethral sigmoidostomy or ileostomy	**Lactic acidosis**	**(RTA) I**
4. Cholestyramine		
	Massive rhabdomyolysis	**Hypoaldosteronism**
Renal		
1. Renal tubular acidosis (RTA) type II	**Ingestion**	**Potassium-sparing diuretics**
2. Carbonic anhydrase inhibitors (acetazalomide)	1. Salicylates	
	2. Hyperalimentation fluids if acetate or lactate is not added	**Posthypercapneic metabolic acidosis after correction of chronic respiratory alkalosis**

- *Ketoacidosis:* Diabetes mellitus, alcoholism, starvation.
- *Lactic acidosis:* Respiratory or circulatory failure, drugs and toxins, hereditary disorders, septic shock. It can be associated with other disease states, such as leukemia, pancreatitis, bacterial infection, and uncontrolled diabetes mellitus.
- *Poisoning and drug toxicity:* Salicylates, methanol, ethylene glycol, ammonium chloride.
- *Loss of alkali:* Draining wounds (e.g., pancreatic fistulas), diarrhea, ureterostomy.

Diagnostic Tests

1. **ABG values:** Determine pH (usually <7.35) and degree of respiratory compensation as reflected by $Paco_2$, which usually is <35 mm Hg.
2. **Serum bicarbonate:** Determines presence of metabolic acidosis (HCO_3^- <22 mEq/L).
3. **Serum electrolytes:** Elevated potassium may be present because of the exchange of intracellular potassium for hydrogen ions in the body's attempt to normalize acid-base environment.
   - *Anion gap:* In attempting to identify the cause of metabolic acidosis, an analysis of serum electrolytes to detect anion gap may be helpful. Anion gap reflects unmeasureable anions present in plasma and is calculated by subtracting the sum of chloride and sodium bicarbonate from the amount of plasma sodium concentration.

   Anion gap = Na^+ minus (Cl^- + HCO_3^-).

4. **ECG:** Detects dysrhythmias caused by hyperkalemia. Changes seen with hyperkalemia include peaked T waves, depressed ST segment, decreased size of R waves, decrease or absence of P waves, and widened QRS complex. Acidosis can cause nonspecific ECG changes.

Collaborative Management

1. **Sodium bicarbonate** ($NaHCO_3$): Usually indicated when arterial pH is ≤7.2. The usual mode of delivery is IV drip: 2-3 ampules (44.5 mEq/ampule) in 1000 ml 5 percent dex-

Anion Gap

Anion Gap Type	Values	Causes
Normal anion gap	12 ($\pm$2) mEq/L	Diarrhea, renal tubular acidosis, or pancreatic fistula causing a direct loss of HCO_3^-; addition of chloride-containing acids.
Increased anion gap	>14 mEq/L	Lactic acidosis, uremia, diabetic ketoacidosis (DKA), or salicylate and methanol toxicity, resulting in accumulation of nonvolatile acids with decrease in HCO_3^-.

For more information about anion gap, see Chapter 5.

trose in water (D_5W), although $NaHCO_3$ frequently is given IV push in emergencies. Concentration depends on severity of the acidosis and presence of any serum sodium disorders. $NaHCO_3$ must be given cautiously to avoid metabolic alkalosis and pulmonary edema secondary to the sodium load.

2. **Potassium replacement:** Usually, hyperkalemia is present but a potassium deficit can occur as well. If a potassium deficit exists (K^+ <3.5), it must be corrected before $NaHCO_3$ is administered because when the acidosis is corrected, the potassium shifts back to intracellular spaces. This could result in serum hypokalemia with serious consequences, such as cardiac irritability with fatal dysrhythmias and generalized muscle weakness. See Chapter 8 for more information.

3. **Mechanical ventilation:** If necessary; however, it is important that the patient's compensatory hyperventilation be allowed to continue to prevent acidosis from becoming more severe. Therefore, the respiratory rate on the ventilator should not be set lower than the rate at which the patient has been breathing spontaneously, and the tidal vol-

ume should be large enough to maintain compensatory hyperventilation until the underlying disorder can be resolved.

4. **Treatment of underlying disorder**
   - *Diabetic ketoacidosis:* Insulin and fluids. If acidosis is severe (with a pH of <7.1 or HCO_3^- 6-8 mEq/L), sodium bicarbonate may be necessary.
   - *Alcoholism-related ketoacidosis:* Glucose and saline.
   - *Diarrhea:* Usually occurs in association with other fluid and electrolyte disturbances; correction addresses concurrent imbalances.
   - *Acute renal failure:* Hemodialysis or peritoneal dialysis to restore an adequate level of plasma bicarbonate. (See Chapter 22.)
   - *Renal tubular acidosis:* May require modest amounts (<100 mEq/day) of bicarbonate.
   - *Poisoning and drug toxicity:* Treatment depends on drug ingested or infused. Hemodialysis or peritoneal dialysis may be necessary.
   - *Lactic acidosis:* Correction of underlying disorder. Mortality associated with lactic acidosis is high. Treatment with $NaHCO_3$ is only transiently helpful.

 # Nursing Diagnoses and Interventions

Nursing diagnoses and interventions are specific to the pathophysiologic process. In addition, see "Acute Respiratory Acidosis" . . . for the following: **Sensory-perceptual alterations,** p. 155; **Altered oral mucous membrane** related to abnormal breathing pattern, p. 156; **Sleep pattern disturbance** related to frequent treatments and procedures, p. 157; and **Ineffective family coping** related to stress reaction, p. 157.

Chronic Metabolic Acidosis

Most often, this condition is seen with chronic renal failure in which the kidneys' ability to excrete acids (endogenous and exogenous) is exceeded by acid production and ingestion. The acidosis usually is mild in the initial stage, with HCO_3^- 18-22 mEq/L and a pH of approximately 7.35. Treatment is indicated when serum bicarbonate levels reach 15 mEq/L. Respiratory compensation does occur, but to a limited degree. A modest decrease in $Paco_2$ will be noted on ABG values.

Assessment

1. **Signs and symptoms:** Usually the patient is asymptomatic, although fatigue, malaise, and anorexia may be present in relation to the underlying disease.
2. **History and risk factors:** Chronic renal failure, renal tubular acidosis.

Diagnostic Tests

1. **Arterial blood gas values:** $Paco_2$ will be <35 mm Hg; pH will be <7.40.
2. **Serum bicarbonate:** Will be <22 mEq/L (usually 18-21 mEq/L). With severe acidosis, it will be ≤15 mEq/L.
3. **Serum electrolytes:** Serum calcium level is checked before treatment of acidosis is initiated to prevent tetany induced by hypocalcemia (caused by a decrease in ionized calcium). Serum potassium level should be monitored after acidosis has been corrected to detect hypokalemia, as potassium shifts back into the cells.

Collaborative Management

1. **Alkalizing agents:** For serum bicarbonate levels <15 mEq/L, oral alkali are administered (sodium bicarbonate tablets or sodium citrate—Shohl's solution). They are used cautiously to prevent fluid overload and tetany caused by hypocalcemia. **Note:** Be alert to the possibility of pulmonary edema if oliguria is present and bicarbonate is administered parenterally. Chronic acidosis is of concern in chronic renal failure because the bones are used as a chronic buffer and this contributes to renal bone disease.
2. **Hemodialysis or peritoneal dialysis:** If indicated by chronic renal failure or other disease processes. Uncontrolled acidosis may be an indicator of the need for initiating or increasing dialytic therapy in the chronic renal failure patient.

ndx: Nursing Diagnoses and Interventions

Altered nutrition: Less than body requirements related to decreased intake secondary to fatigue, dietary restrictions, and metallic taste in the mouth (owing to uremic state)
Desired outcome: Patient's weight remains stable.

1. Provide foods that correspond to patient's prescribed diet and preference.
2. Offer small meals and snacks at frequent intervals.
3. Offer oral care often to minimize the metallic taste. Brushing teeth before meals and using mouthwash frequently throughout the day are helpful.
4. Provide hard candy to keep the oral mucosa moist, diminish metallic taste, and supply calories.
5. Monitor hemoglobin and hematocrit levels to determine if anemia may be contributing to patient's fatigue.
6. Provide periods of uninterrupted rest by clustering necessary treatments and procedures. If possible, avoid performing unpleasant or uncomfortable treatments one hour before and after mealtimes.
7. Encourage family members to eat with patient or be present at mealtimes to provide social interaction.

Other nursing diagnoses and interventions are specific to the underlying pathophysiologic process.

Metabolic Alkalosis

Acute Metabolic Alkalosis

This disorder results in an elevated serum bicarbonate >24 mEq/L and a pH >7.40 as a result of hydrogen ion loss or excess alkali intake. A compensatory increase in Pa_{CO_2} (up to 50-60 mm Hg) will be seen. Respiratory compensation is limited because of hypoxia, which develops secondary to decreased alveolar ventilation. The major causes of acute metabolic alkalosis are loss of gastric acid from vomiting or nasogastric (NG) suction, posthypercapnic alkalosis (which occurs when chronic CO_2 retention is corrected rapidly), excessive sodium bicarbonate administration (i.e., overcorrection of a metabolic acidosis), and thiazide diuretic therapy.

Assessment

1. **Signs and symptoms:** Muscular weakness, neuromuscular instability and hyporeflexia secondary to accompanying hypokalemia. Decrease in GI tract motility may result in an ileus. Severe alkalosis can result in signs of neuromuscular excitability as well as apathy, confusion, and stupor.
2. **Electrocardiogram (ECG) findings:** Numerous types of atrial-ventricular dysrhythmias as a result of the cardiac irritability occurring with hypokalemia; U waves.
3. **History and risk factors** (see accompanying box):
   - *Clinical circumstances associated with volume/chloride depletion:* Vomiting or gastric drainage.
   - *Posthypercapneic alkalosis.*
   - *Excessive alkali intake:* May be iatrogenic from overcorrection of metabolic acidosis (frequently seen during cardiopulmonary resuscitation [CPR]). Excessive ingestion

Potential Causes of Metabolic Alkalosis

H^+ Loss

1. Gastrointestinal
   - Loss of gastric secretions (NG suctioning or vomiting)*
   - Villous adenoma
   - Congenital chloridorrhea
2. Renal
   - Diuretics (especially *loop* and thiazides*)
   - Mineralocorticoid excess*
   - Post chronic hypocapnia
   - Carbenicillin/penicillin derivation
   - Hypercalcemia/hypoparathyroidism
3. H^+ shift into the cells
   - Hypokalemia*
   - Carbohydrate refeeding after starvation

HCO_3^- Retention

1. Administration of bicarbonate or bicarbonate precursors
2. Massive blood transfusion
3. Milk-alkali syndrome

Contraction Alkalosis

Diuretics
Cystic fibrosis

*Most common causes.

of sodium bicarbonate (e.g., Alka-Seltzer) or calcium carbonate (e.g., Tums, Rolaids) is another potential cause.
- *Acute, aggressive thiazide diuretic therapy.*

Diagnostic Tests

1. **Arterial blood gas (ABG) values:** Determine severity of alkalosis and response to therapy. The pH will be >7.40.
2. **Serum bicarbonate:** Values will be elevated to >26 mEq/L.

3. **Serum electrolytes:** Usually, serum potassium will be low (<4.0 mEq/L) as will serum chloride (<95 mEq/L). Although the relationship between metabolic alkalosis and potassium is not completely understood, alkalosis and hypokalemia often occur together.
4. **ECG:** To assess for dysrhythmias, especially if profound hypokalemia or alkalosis is present.

Collaborative Management

Management will depend on the underlying disorder. Mild or moderate metabolic alkalosis usually does not require specific therapeutic interventions.

1. **Saline infusion:** Normal saline infusion may correct volume (chloride) deficit in patients with alkalosis secondary to gastric losses. Metabolic alkalosis is difficult to correct if hypovolemia and chloride deficit are not corrected.
2. **Potassium chloride (KCl):** Indicated for patients with low potassium levels. KCl is preferred over other potassium salts because chloride losses can be replaced simultaneously.
3. **Sodium and potassium chloride:** Effective for posthypercapneic alkalosis, which occurs when chronic CO_2 retention is corrected rapidly (e.g., *via* mechanical ventilation). If adequate amounts of chloride and potassium are not available, renal excretion of excess bicarbonate is impaired and metabolic alkalosis continues.
4. **Histamine H_2-receptor antagonists (e.g., cimetidine, ranitidine, and famotidine):** Reduce production of gastric hydrochloric acid (HCl) and therefore are useful in preventing or decreasing the metabolic alkalosis that can occur with gastric suctioning.
5. **Carbonic anhydrase inhibitors:** Acetazolamide (Diamox) is especially useful for correcting metabolic alkalosis for patients who cannot tolerate rapid volume expansion (e.g., individuals with CHF). It can be given orally or intravenously. Acetazolamide causes a large increase in renal secretion of bicarbonate ion (HCO_3^-) and K^+, and therefore it may be necessary to supplement potassium before giving the drug.

6. **Acidifying agents:** Severe metabolic alkalosis (pH of
   >7.60 and HCO_3^- 40–45 mEq/L) may require treatment
   with acidifying agents such as dilute hydrochloride acid,
   ammonium chloride, or argenine hydrochloride. Because
   of their serious side effects, these medications are not used
   frequently.

Nursing Diagnoses and Interventions

Nursing diagnoses and interventions are specific to the underlying pathophysiologic process. In addition, the following may ap-
ply.
Decreased cardiac output related to electrical factors (risk of
dysrhythmias) secondary to metabolic alkalosis induced by gastric suctioning or potassium–wasting diuretics
Desired outcome: ECG reveals a normal tracing; pH is ≤7.45.

1. Monitor laboratory values, especially pH and serum carbon dioxide (CO_2) to determine patient's response to therapy. Notify MD if there are significant changes or lack of
   response to treatment.
2. Monitor ECG for the presence of dysrhythmias. Assess
   apical and radial pulses simultaneously when evaluating
   cardiac rate and rhythm to detect pulse deficit. Notify MD
   of any changes in cardiac rate and rhythm.
3. Monitor potassium levels, especially in patients receiving
   digitalis preparations. (Recall that hypokalemia frequently
   coexists with metabolic alkalosis.) Notify MD if potassium
   levels drop to <3.5 mEq/L. Hypokalemia sensitizes patients to the cardiotoxic effect of digitalis.
4. Use isotonic saline solutions to irrigate gastric tubes. Water is not recommended for irrigation because it can cause
   a washout of electrolytes.
5. If the patient is permitted to have ice chips, administer
   limited quantities to avoid washing electrolytes from the
   patient's stomach. Total volume of ice consumed over a
   shift frequently is underestimated. Determine the volume
   of a specific number of ice cubes or the quantity of
   crushed ice by melting and measuring. Establish the volume of fluid the patient may consume each shift. Document the volume consumed in ml or ounces, not by the
   number of cubes.

6. Measure and document the amount of fluid removed by suction.
7. Weigh patient daily to determine fluid volume status.
8. Administer histamine H_2^- receptor antagonist (e.g., ranitidine) as prescribed to block hydrochloride secretion or famotidine by the stomach, thus lessening systemic metabolic alkalosis.
9. Monitor and record patient's rate and depth of respirations. Diuretic-induced metabolic alkalosis eliminates the force acidemia normally would exert to sustain the respiratory drive, resulting in the potential for compromised respirations. **Note:** This disorder usually is not seen in the alert patient.

Chronic Metabolic Alkalosis

Chronic metabolic alkalosis results in a pH >7.45. $Paco_2$ will be elevated (>45 mm Hg) to compensate for the loss of hydrogen ion (H^+) or excess serum HCO_3^-. There are three clinical situations in which this can occur: (1) abnormalities in the kidneys' excretion of HCO_3^- related to a mineralcorticoid effect; (2) loss of H^+ through the GI tract; and (3) diuretic therapy.

Assessment

1. **Signs and symptoms:** Patient may be asymptomatic. With severe potassium depletion and profound alkalosis, patient may experience weakness, neuromuscular instability, and decrease in GI tract motility, which can result in ileus.
2. **ECG findings:** Frequent premature ventricular contractions (PVCs) or U waves with hypokalemia and alkalosis.
3. **History and risk factors**
   - *Diuretic use:* Thiazide diuretics cause a loss of chloride, potassium, and hydrogen ions. Massive depletion of potassium stores with loss of up to 1000 mEq, which is one third of total body potassium, may occur, causing profound hypokalemia ($K^+ \leq 2.0$ mEq).
   - *Hyperadrenocorticism:* Cushing's syndrome, primary aldosteronism. Not a chloride deficit but a chronic loss of potassium, which can lead to total body depletion

of potassium with profound hypokalemia (K^+ ≤2.0 mEq/L).

- *Chronic vomiting or chronic GI losses through gastric suction.*
- *Milk alkali syndrome:* An infrequent cause of metabolic alkalosis. Hypercalcemic nephropathy and alkalosis develop secondary to excessive intake of absorbable alkali.

Diagnostic Tests

1. **ABG values:** Determine severity of acid-base imbalance. $Paco_2$ will be increased (>45 mm Hg) and pH will be >7.40.
2. **Serum bicarbonate:** Will be >26 mEq/L.
3. **Serum electrolytes:** Usually, potassium will be profoundly low (may be ≤2.0 mEq/L). Chloride may be <95 mEq/L and magnesium may be <1.5 mEq/L. Hypomagnesemia may contribute to irritability of the myocardium.

Collaborative Management

The goal is to correct the underlying acid-base disorder *via* the following interventions.

1. **Fluid management:** If volume depletion exists, normal saline infusions are given.
2. **Potassium replacement:** If a chloride deficit also is present, potassium chloride is the drug of choice. If a chloride deficit does not exist, other potassium salts are acceptable.

- *IV potassium:* If the patient is on a cardiac monitor, up to 20 mEq/hour of potassium chloride is given for serious hypokalemia. Concentrated doses of KCl (>40 mEq/L) require administration through a central venous line because of blood vessel irritation.
- *Oral potassium:* Tastes *very* unpleasant. 15 mEq per glass is all most patients can tolerate, with a maximum daily dose of 60-80 mEq. Slow-release potassium tablets are an acceptable form of KCl. All forms of KCl may be irritating to gastric or intestinal mucosa.
- *Dietary:* Normal diet contains 3 g or 75 mEq of potassium, but not in the form of potassium chloride. Dietary

supplementation of potassium is not effective if a concurrent chloride deficit is also present.

3. **Potassium-sparing diuretics:** May be added to treatment if thiazide diuretics are the cause of hypokalemia and metabolic alkalosis.

4. **Identify and correct cause of hyperadrenocorticism.**

Nursing Diagnoses and Interventions

Knowledge deficit: Necessary precautions for taking thiazide diuretics

Desired outcome: Patient verbalizes knowledge about thiazide diuretics and the necessary precautions that must be taken.

1. Provide patient and significant others with the following information about the prescribed thiazide diuretic: name, purpose, dosage, precautions, and potential side effects.

2. Stress the importance of taking only the prescribed dose, as higher concentrations of the medication increase the risk of hypokalemia and alkalosis.

3. Explain that diets high in sodium increase the risk of alkalosis and hypokalemia, necessitating restrictions of sodium as prescribed.

4. If KCl supplements are prescribed, teach patient the following:
   - Oral potassium has an unpleasant taste and is most palatable when mixed with orange juice or tomato juice.
   - Slow-release tablets should not be chewed.
   - Both of the above can irritate the stomach and should be taken with meals.
   - Although many foods contain potassium, they should not be used as a substitute for the potassium chloride supplements prescribed by the patient's physician.

For other nursing diagnoses and interventions, see "Acute Metabolic Alkalosis" for the following: **Decreased cardiac output** related to electrical factors (risk of dysrhythmias) secondary to metabolic alkalosis induced by gastric suctioning or potassium–wasting diuretics, p 178.

Mixed Acid-Base Disorders

17

Mixed Acid-Base Disorders

A mixed acid-base disturbance occurs when two or more simple acid-base disorders are present at the same time. The effect of a mixed acid-base disturbance on the pH depends on both the specific disorders involved and their severity. If a mixed disorder involves two types of acidosis, a larger drop in pH can be expected than would occur if a mixed acidosis-alkalosis disorder were present. When two opposing disorders (i.e., an acidosis and an alkalosis) co-occur, the pH will be determined by the predominant disorder. In some cases, the pH will be normal in the presence of a mixed acid-base disorder (see Table 17-1).

Case Study One

The patient has a history of chronic obstructive pulmonary disease (COPD) with carbon dioxide (CO_2) retention and is admitted after 3 days of diarrhea. The patient's normal response to an increased $Paco_2$ (respiratory acidosis) is a compensatory increase in serum bicarbonate ion (HCO_3^-).

Values

pH	$Paco_2$	HCO_3^-
7.23	65 mm Hg	29 mEq/L

Table 17-1   Mixed acid-base disorders

Types	Examples
Metabolic acidosis and metabolic acidosis	Renal failure, diarrhea
Acute respiratory acidosis and chronic respiratory acidosis	Pneumonia, emphysema
Metabolic acidosis and metabolic alkalosis	Diabetic ketoacidosis, vomiting
Metabolic acidosis and respiratory acidosis	Lactic acidosis, respiratory arrest
Metabolic acidosis and respiratory alkalosis	Ethylene glycol ingestion, pneumonia
Metabolic alkalosis and respiratory acidosis	Gastric suction, sedative overdose
Metabolic alkalosis and respiratory alkalosis	Diuretic use, hepatic failure

Evaluation

The loss of bicarbonate secondary to the diarrhea leads to a decreased HCO_3^- with a concomitant metabolic acidosis. Although the HCO_3^- remains higher than normal, it is lower than would be expected for this patient. These values, with the patient's history, reflect a mixed acid-base disorder: respiratory acidosis and metabolic acidosis.

Case Study Two

The patient is admitted with a history of cirrhosis and prolonged diarrhea.

Values

pH	Paco$_2$	Na$^+$	K$^+$	Cl$^-$	HCO$_3^-$	Anion Gap
7.38	28	138	2.9	115	13	10

Anion gap determination: $138 - (115 + 13) = 10$ where the terms correspond to Na^+, Cl^-, HCO_3^-

Evaluation

Cirrhosis stimulates the respiratory center, resulting in respiratory alkalosis. Prolonged diarrhea has resulted in the loss of HCO_3^-, leading to metabolic acidosis with normal anion gap. Over time, respiratory alkalosis can result in a compensatory decrease in serum HCO_3^-, but normally serum HCO_3^- does not decrease below 16 mEq/L as a compensatory measure. Therefore these values, along with the patient's history, reflect a mixed acid-base disorder: respiratory alkalosis and metabolic acidosis. The pH is in the normal range because the opposing disorders, respiratory alkalosis, and metabolic acidosis, have "balanced" each other.

Case Study Three

The patient is an 80-year-old male who is 3 days post-transurethral resection, with nausea, slight confusion, and a temperature of 38.9°C (102°F).

Values

pH	Pa_{CO_2}	Na^+	K^+	Cl^-	HCO_3^-	anion gap
7.41	30	140	3.7	95	19	26

Anion gap determination: $Na^+ - (Cl^- + HCO_3^-) = 140 - (95 + 19) = 26$

Evaluation

Sepsis-induced stimulation of the respiratory center leads to respiratory alkalosis. Metabolic acidosis results from lactic acid production caused by vasodilatation from septic shock. The presence of an increased anion gap (>14) signals the addition of nonvolatile acids to the system, indicating that the decreased HCO_3^- is not a renal compensatory response to the respiratory alkalosis. These values, along with the patient's history, reflect a mixed acid-base disorder: respiratory alkalosis and anion gap metabolic acidosis. **Note:** Respiratory alkalosis is often an early, subtle sign of the onset of serious illness or complication in a hospitalized patient.

Case Study Four

Twenty minutes ago the patient experienced a cardiac arrest secondary to ventricular dysrhythmias. The patient was given two ampules of sodium bicarbonate and is being ventilated manually at a rate of 24 breaths per minute.

Values

pH	Pa_{CO_2}	HCO_3^-
7.65	28	36

Evaluation

The elevated serum HCO_3^- is a result of overadministration of sodium bicarbonate during resuscitation and is the cause of the metabolic alkalosis. The respiratory alkalosis that *is* present has occurred because of the manual hyperventilation. Based on the patient's history and laboratory values, the patient has a mixed acid-base disorder: metabolic alkalosis and respiratory alkalosis.

Routine administration of sodium bicarbonate is no longer recommended for cardiac arrest.

19-25 ⎤ ⎤ -7/7
26-01 ⎦ ⎬ 7/7 = 14/7
2/day lees

CLINICAL CONDITIONS ASSOCIATED WITH FLUID, ELECTROLYTE, AND ACID-BASE IMBALANCE

Gastrointestinal Disorders 18

As stated in Chapter 3, the gastrointestinal (GI) tract plays an important role in maintaining fluid and electrolyte balance because in health it is the primary site of fluid and electrolyte gain. Approximately 1.5–2.0 L of fluid are gained each day through the consumption of fluids and solid food. Additionally, 6–8 L of fluid are secreted into and reabsorbed out of the GI tract daily, equaling approximately half of the extracellular fluid (ECF) volume. Despite this large volume, the GI tract contributes minimally to normal fluid loss (approximately 100–200 ml/day). In disease, however, the GI tract becomes the most common site of abnormal fluid and electrolyte loss, potentially resulting in profound fluid and electrolyte imbalance.

The composition of the GI secretions varies with the location within the GI tract (Table 18-1). Therefore, the nature of the fluid and electrolyte imbalance will vary with the type of fluid lost. GI fluids include saliva and bile, as well as gastric, pancreatic, and intestinal secretions. GI disorders causing fluid and electrolyte loss may be differentiated into loss of upper GI contents and loss of lower GI contents.

Loss of Upper Gastrointestinal Contents

Upper GI secretions include saliva and gastric juices. Losses may occur due to problems such as vomiting and procedures such as gastric suction. See the box on p. 191 for potential causes of vomiting.

Table 18-1   Volume and composition of gastrointestinal secretions*

Secretion	Liter/24°	Na$^+$ mEq/L	K$^+$ mEq/L	Cl$^-$ mEq/L	HCO$_3$$^-$ mEq/L
Saliva	1	40	15	30	0
Gastric juice	1-2	40	7	100	0
Pancreatic juice	1-2	130	7	60	100
Bile	1	150	7	80	30
Intestinal secretions	1-2	140	5	variable	variable

*Values are approximate

Potential Causes of Vomiting

- Gastrointestinal infection
- Inner ear infection
- Certain medications (e.g., chemotherapy)
- Pregnancy
- Small bowel obstruction
- Pyloric stenosis
- Uremia
- Binge-purge syndrome
- Pancreatitis
- Hepatitis
- Diabetic ketoacidosis

Saliva

Approximately 1 L of saliva is produced each day. Saliva begins the digestive process by initiating the breakdown of starches. In addition, it lubricates food, facilitating swallowing. Food and saliva move through the esophagus to the stomach by means of peristalsis (rhythmic contractions). Once in the stomach, the food and saliva are exposed to the acidic secretions found there (see "Gastric Juices," below). Abnormal loss of saliva may occur in individuals who are unable to swallow their oral secretions (e.g., those who are comatose).

Gastric Juices

Approximately 1-2 L of gastric juices are produced daily and contain hydrochloric acid (HCl), which aids digestion by breaking down food; the enzyme pepsin, which initiates digestion of proteins; and intrinsic factor, which facilitates the absorption of vitamin B_{12} in the ileum.

Only alcohol and a limited amount of water are absorbed from the stomach. Most of the stomach contents moves by peristalsis into the small intestine. Although the fluid and electrolyte content of food is quite variable, gastric contents mix and become similar in concentration to the ECF owing to osmotic shifts of water into and out of the stomach. Losses from the upper GI tract (above the pylorus) are essentially isotonic and rich in sodium, potassium, chloride, and hydrogen (see Table 18-1).

Gastric Suction

Gastric suction, whether *via* a nasogastric or orogastric tube, is a common medical procedure used to decompress the stomach. Removal of gastric contents may lead to multiple fluid and electrolyte imbalances and requires adequate parenteral replacement. This may be accomplished by administering an IV solution developed specifically for gastric replacement (e.g., Isolyte G made by McGaw) or customizing a solution to meet the individual patient's needs, based on serum electrolyte levels. The following are nursing considerations that are important for minimizing electrolyte imbalance with gastric suction:

1. **Give patient nothing by mouth (NPO).**
2. **Avoid giving ice by mouth or irrigating the catheter with plain water** as these actions will increase the loss of electrolytes due to "wash out." If patients are allowed ice chips, give small amounts (less than 1 oz) hourly.
3. **Provide frequent oral care** to minimize thirst and maximize comfort.
4. **Irrigate gastric tube with normal saline (isotonic NaCl solution) only.** If the catheter is irrigated and an equal amount is not withdrawn and discarded, the extra irrigant should be added to the intake record to avoid overestimation of the fluid loss.

Potential Fluid, Electrolyte, and Acid Base Disturbances with Loss of Upper Gastrointestinal Contents

1. **Hypovolemia** due to abnormal fluid loss. (See Chapter 6.)
2. **Hyponatremia** due to loss of sodium-rich fluids with inadequate electrolyte replacement; and/or due to ADH and thirst-induced retention of water. (See Chapter 7.)
3. **Hypokalemia** due to loss of potassium-rich fluids with inadequate replacement. Increased production of aldosterone secondary to hypovolemia will contribute to the develop-

ment of hypokalemia owing to increased renal losses. Remember that aldosterone causes both an increased retention of sodium and increased excretion of potassium. (See Chapter 8.)

4. **Hypomagnesemia** due to prolonged loss of upper GI fluids with inadequate replacement. (See Chapter 11.)
5. **Metabolic alkalosis** due to loss of fluids rich in chloride and hydrogen. Hypovolemia contributes to the development and perpetuation of metabolic alkalosis due to volume-induced conservation of sodium bicarbonate ($NaHCO_3$). (See Chapter 16.)

Loss of Lower Gastrointestinal Contents

The small intestines are the primary site of nutrient, electrolyte, and water absorption. Approximately 8 L of fluid enter the small intestines from the upper GI tract daily, of which 75% is absorbed (and returned to the ECF). The colon receives only 1–2 L of fluid from the ileum; of this, normally all are absorbed except 100–200 ml of water and a small quantity of electrolytes.

Losses from the lower GI tract (below the pylorus) are generally isotonic and rich in sodium, potassium, and bicarbonate. Lower GI contents may be lost through diarrhea, intestinal fistulas, or intestinal resection. Abnormal losses from the small intestines of as much as 2000 ml/day may occur with the creation of a new ileostomy or with short bowel syndrome. Although the loss of water and electrolytes remains greater than that with normal stool, over time ileostomy output decreases to only 300–500 ml/day. Fistulas (an abnormal passage from the bowel to the skin) also may result in the loss of several liters of intestinal fluid daily. Diarrhea, however, remains the most common cause of lower GI fluid loss, especially in children. In developed countries diarrhea accounts for a significant percentage of pediatric hospital admissions and clinic visits. In underdeveloped nations, diarrhea is a major cause of infant deaths. (See "Diarrhea," below, and box on p. 194).

Vomiting can contribute to lower GI fluid loss because both gastric and duodenal contents may be lost. Losses from both the upper and lower GI tract also can occur with bowel obstruction.

Potential Causes of Diarrhea

Osmotic Diarrhea
- Certain medications (e.g., lactulose, sorbitol)
- Malabsorption or maldigestion syndromes

Secretory Diarrhea
- GI infection
- Inflammatory bowel disease
- Emotional stress
- Pancreatic insufficiency
- Intestinal obstruction
- Abuse of laxatives (e.g., bisacodyl, castor oil)
- Carcinoma

Acid-base balance usually is maintained when both gastric and duodenal fluids are lost, because a loss of both hydrogen (acid) and bicarbonate (base) occurs.

Lower GI secretions include bile, pancreatic juice, and intestinal secretions (succus entericus).

Pancreatic Juice

Approximately 1-2 L of pancreatic juice are secreted each day. Pancreatic juice is high in bicarbonate, which neutralizes the acidic gastric contents as they enter the duodenum. It also contains enzymes that aid in the digestion of protein (trypsin), starches (amylase), and fats (lipase).

Bile

Bile is produced by the liver and stored in the gallbladder. Water and electrolytes are continuously reabsorbed by the gallbladder mucosa so that the bile released into the duodenum may be five to ten times more concentrated than the bile produced by the liver. The liver produces approximately 1 L of bile per day. Bile provides a means of excreting bilirubin (a breakdown product of hemoglobin) and aids in the digestion of fats *via* emulsification by bile salts. In addition to bilirubin and bile salts, bile contains water, sodium, potassium, calcium, bicarbonate, cholesterol, and lecithin.

Intestinal Secretions

In addition to bile and pancreatic juice, the intestines contain secretions produced by the intestinal glands. These glands secrete mucus, which helps protect the intestinal mucosa, hormones (e.g., secretin), electrolytes, and digestive enzymes. Approximately 1-2 L of intestinal gland secretions are produced each day. The secretion of isotonic intestinal fluids may increase dramatically in certain diseases such as cholera and other intestinal infections, after administration of certain medications such as laxatives, and with bowel obstruction (see below).

Diarrhea

Diarrhea is defined as an increased loss of fluid and electrolytes *via* the stool. The causes of diarrhea are divided into two main categories: (1) those causing osmotic diarrhea and (2) those causing secretory diarrhea. *Osmotic diarrhea* occurs when poorly absorbable solutes are present in the colon. The unabsorbed solutes create an osmotic gradient for water to move from the ECF into the lumen of the bowel. Additionally, water that normally would be reabsorbed from the bowel remains in the lumen. This is the means by which sorbitol and lactulose induce diarrhea. Malabsorption or maldigestion of carbohydrates also will result in osmotic diarrhea because bacteria in the colon convert unabsorbed carbohydrates to organic acids. These organic acids create an osmotic gradient favoring the production of liquid stools. Osmotic diarrhea usually stops within 24–48 hours of fasting.

Water and electrolytes are both secreted into and reabsorbed from the lumen of the bowel. Under normal conditions there is net reabsorption, minimizing the volume of the stool. *Secretory diarrhea* develops when there is either increased secretion or decreased reabsorption of water and electrolytes. Unlike osmotic diarrhea, secretory diarrhea does not cease with fasting and is characterized by large losses of water and electrolytes. Bacterial infections cause secretory diarrhea by irritating the bowel mucosa and causing increased secretion of water and electrolytes. The diarrhea that occurs with inflammatory bowel diseases (ulcerative colitis and Crohn's disease) is believed to be the result of inflammation of the bowel wall, which causes both an increase in the secretion and decrease in reabsorption. The individual with inflammatory bowel disease may pass more than five stools per day, causing both physical and emotional debilitation.

Bowel Obstruction

The type and extent of fluid and electrolyte imbalance that occurs with bowel obstruction will depend on the location of the obstruction and its duration. The longer the bowel is obstructed, the more profound the fluid and electrolyte imbalance. Lower GI loss occurs because of sequestering of fluid in the distended bowel. Several liters of fluid may collect in the intestinal lumen, leading to a dramatic increase in lumen pressure and eventual damage to the intestinal mucosa. Peritonitis may then occur if bacteria enter the peritoneal cavity through the damaged intestinal wall. The fluid sequestered in the bowel is inaccessible to the ECF, creating a separate third space. Peritonitis also causes a shift of fluid into the temporarily inaccessible third space. Normally the peritoneum aids in the rapid transport of fluid from the peritoneal cavity to the circulation. When the peritoneum becomes damaged or inflamed, fluid and electrolytes collect in the peritoneal cavity. The loss of ECF into an inaccessible third space causes a reduction in effective circulating volume, which stimulates both thirst and release of ADH, with the retention of water. These two factors lead to the eventual development of *dilutional hyponatremia*. Upper GI loss can occur with bowel obstruction owing to the increased stimulus to vomit.

Potential Fluid, Electrolyte, and Acid-Base Disturbances with Loss of Lower Gastrointestinal Contents

1. **Hypovolemia** due to abnormal fluid loss. (See Chapter 6.)
2. **Hyponatremia** due to loss of sodium-rich fluids with inadequate electrolyte replacement; or due to thirst and ADH–induced retention of water. (See Chapter 7.)
3. **Hypokalemia** due to loss of potassium-rich fluids, com-

bined with inadequate replacement. (See Chapter 8.)

4. **Hypomagnesemia** due to abnormal fluid loss. (See Chapter 11.) Typically, hypomagnesemia occurs only with prolonged loss of GI fluids, such as with ulcerative colitis.

5. **Metabolic acidosis** due to loss of fluids rich in bicarbonate. (See Chapter 15.)

Surgical Disturbances 19

Disturbances in fluid and electrolyte balance are common in the surgical patient owing to a combination of factors that occur preoperatively, intraoperatively, and postoperatively.

Preoperative Factors

1. **Preexisting conditions** such as diabetes mellitus, hypertension, liver disease, or renal insufficiency, which may be aggravated by the stress of surgery. (See Chapters 20, 22, and 24.)
2. **Diagnostic procedures** such as arteriogram or intravenous pyelogram (IVP) that require administration of intravenous dyes, which may cause inappropriate urinary excretion of water and electrolytes owing to the osmotic diuresis effect.
3. **Administration of medications** such as steroids or diuretics, which may affect the excretion of water and electrolytes.
4. **Surgical preparations** such as enemas or laxatives, which may act to increase fluid loss from the GI tract. (See Chapter 18.)
5. **Medical management of preexisting conditions.** Examples include gastric suction and gastric lavage.
6. **Preoperative fluid restriction** (i.e., "NPO after midnight"). During an average 6-hour period of fluid restriction, the healthy patient loses approximately 300-500 ml of fluid owing to normal fluid loss. Fluid loss may be increased greatly if the patient is experiencing abnormal fluid loss or fever.

Intraoperative Factors

1. **Induction of anesthesia,** which may lead to the development of hypotension in the patient with preoperative hypovolemia owing to the loss of compensatory mechanisms such as tachycardia or vasoconstriction.
2. **Abnormal blood loss** related to preoperative trauma or the surgical procedure itself.
3. **Abnormal loss of extracellular fluid (ECF) into a third space,** for example, the loss of ECF into the wall and lumen of the bowel during bowel surgery. This fluid is temporarily unavailable either to the intracellular fluid (ICF) or ECF, hence it is termed "third-space fluid." Loss of ECF also occurs when intravascular volume is lost into a nonequilibrating space, for example, bleeding into a fractured hip.
4. **Loss of fluid from the surgical wound.** This usually is of concern with large wounds and prolonged operative procedures.

Note: All of the above factors relate to fluid volume. (See Chapter 6.)

Postoperative Factors

1. **Stress of surgery and postoperative pain,** which leads to an increased release of antidiuretic hormone (ADH) by the posterior pituitary gland and an increased release of adrenocorticotropic hormone (ACTH) by the anterior pituitary gland. Increased ADH results in retention of water by the kidneys. Excessive production may lead to the development of hyponatremia (See Chapter 7). ACTH acts on the adrenal cortex to cause an increase in the release of aldosterone and hydrocortisone. Both aldosterone and hydrocortisone lead to an increased retention of sodium and water and an increased excretion of potassium by the kidneys. The combined effects of these hormones may result in postoperative fluid retention lasting up to 48-72 hours (see Chapter 6).
2. **Increase in tissue catabolism** (breakdown) secondary to tissue trauma, which causes the patient to produce a

greater than normal amount of water from oxidation. (See Chapter 6.)

3. **Reduction in effective circulating volume (ECV),** which stimulates production of ADH and aldosterone. Potential causes include bleeding, fluid loss from the surgical wound, abnormal sequestration of fluid (i.e., third space shift), draining fistulas, gastric suction, vomiting, and increased insensible fluid loss from fever. (See Chapter 6.)

4. **Risk or presence of postoperative ileus,** which may restrict the patient's ability to take oral fluids and necessitate gastric suction. (See Chapter 18.)

5. **Hyperkalemia,** which may occur during the immediate postoperative period, due to the release of intracellular potassium secondary to tissue trauma. (See Chapter 8.)

6. **Metabolic acidosis,** which may occur due to an abnormal production of lactic acid in the hypotensive patient who experiences tissue hypoxia. (See Chapter 15.)

7. **Respiratory acidosis,** which may develop due to inadequate ventilation secondary to respiratory depression from anesthesia or pain medication, splinting of the operative site, or restriction to bed, increasing the risk of atelectasis or pneumonia, especially in the patient with COPD. (See Chapter 13.)

8. **Fluid, electrolyte, and acid-base disturbances,** which may occur with abnormal loss of GI fluids due to vomiting, diarrhea, and gastric or intestinal suctioning. (See Chapter 18.)

Endocrinologic Disorders

20

Diabetic Ketoacidosis (DKA)

DKA occurs as a result of an absolute or relative insulin deficiency. An absolute lack of insulin occurs in the individual with newly diagnosed Type I (insulin-dependent) diabetes or in the patient with diabetes who stops taking insulin; whereas a relative insulin deficiency occurs in the patient with diabetes who suddenly has an increased insulin need, usually owing to some form of physical or emotional stress such as infection, surgery, or an acute illness. Insulin deficiency leads to hyperglycemia due to decreased glucose utilization by the cells and increased hepatic glucose production, and to ketonemia (increased ketones in the blood) owing to altered fat metabolism with increased production of ketones (acetone, acetoacetic acid, and beta-hydroxybutyric acid). Hyperglycemia and ketonemia in turn lead to a combination of potentially life-threatening fluid and electrolyte imbalances.

Both hyperglycemia and ketonemia contribute to the development of hyperosmolality with movement of water out of the cells. The neurologic changes seen in DKA are the result of intracellular dehydration within the central nervous system. At the same time, the presence of ketones and excess glucose in the urine causes an osmotic diuresis, with loss of water and electrolytes in the urine. This polyuria may lead to profound fluid volume deficit and shock and contributes to the development of hypokalemia, hypophosphatemia, and hypomagnesemia.

Despite the loss of substantial quantities of electrolytes in the urine, patients initially may present with normal or elevated levels of the major intracellular electrolytes (e.g., potassium, magnesium, and phosphorus). This occurs in part because of increased tissue catabolism (breakdown) with the release of intra-cellular electrolytes. In addition, insulin deficiency results in a decreased movement of potassium into the cell, and acidosis causes an increased movement of potassium out of the cell.

Actual deficiencies of potassium, phosphorus, and magnesium become apparent only with treatment as these electrolytes move back into the cells.

Metabolic acidosis occurs with ketosis due to the increased production of organic acids (ketoacids). The situation may be complicated further by the development of lactic acidosis if dehydration leads to decreased tissue perfusion. Kussmaul's respirations are an attempt by the lungs to reduce the acid load by blowing off excess carbon dioxide.

Potential Fluid, Electrolyte, and Acid-Base Disturbances

1. **Fluid volume deficit** due to polyuria secondary to hyperglycemia and ketonemia. Initially, hypovolemia is treated with isotonic saline (0.9% NaCl) administered at a rapid rate. Subsequent volume replacement is with 0.45% NaCl solution, which more closely approximates the fluid loss. Once the blood glucose level falls to 250–300 mg/dl, dextrose-containing solutions are used (e.g., 5% dextrose in 0.45% NaCl or 5% dextrose in 0.225% NaCl).

2. **Hyponatremia** due to the osmotic shift of water out of the cells (pseudohyponatremia). (See Chapter 7.)

3. **Hypernatremia** due to dehydration secondary to osmotic diuresis with the loss of free water (i.e., water is lost in excess of electrolytes). Hypernatremia is corrected with administration of hypotonic IV fluids. (See Chapter 7.)

4. **Hyperkalemia** (initially) due to movement of potassium out of the cell secondary to tissue catabolism, acidosis, and insulin deficiency. (See Chapter 8.)

5. **Hyperphosphatemia** (initially) due to the movement of phosphorus out of the cell secondary to tissue catabolism. (See Chapter 10.)

6. **Hypokalemia** due to the loss of potassium secondary to osmotic diuresis and the movement of potassium back into the cell occurring with the administration of insulin and

correction of acidosis. Potassium levels may drop precipitously with treatment of DKA, requiring frequent monitoring and aggressive potassium replacement. (See Chapter 8.)

7. **Hypophosphatemia and hypomagnesemia** due to the loss of these electrolytes secondary to osmotic diuresis and repair of the tissue with treatment. Hypophosphatemia is corrected by replacing a portion of the potassium deficit with potassium phosphate. (See Chapters 10 and 11.)

8. **Metabolic acidosis** occurring with the abnormal production of ketoacids and lactic acid. Metabolic acidosis usually reverses with the administration of insulin and fluids. Severe acidosis, however, may require treatment with IV sodium bicarbonate. (See Chapter 15.)

Hyperosmolar Hyperglycemic Nonketotic Coma (HHNC)

HHNC is a life-threatening emergency characterized by severe hyperglycemia (blood glucose levels exceed 600 mg/dl and may be as high as 2000 mg/dl) with the absence of significant ketonemia. As with DKA, hyperglycemia causes an osmotic diuresis with loss of electrolytes, including potassium, magnesium, and phosphorus. The diuresis is hypotonic in relation to the electrolytes (i.e., water is lost in excess of sodium and other electrolytes). The combination of hypotonic fluid loss and hyperglycemia leads to serum hyperosmolality. In turn, increased serum osmolality causes a shift of water out of the cells. The net result is a loss of both intracellular fluid (ICF) and extracellular fluid (ECF), with individuals losing up to 25% of their total body water. Neurologic deficits (i.e., slowed mentation, confusion, seizures, or coma) occur as a result of the altered central nervous system (CNS) cell function secondary to cell shrinkage.

As extracellular volume (ECV) decreases, the blood becomes more viscous and its flow is impeded. Thromboemboli are common because of increased blood viscosity, enhanced platelet aggregation and adhesiveness, and patient immobility. Cardiac workload is increased and may lead to myocardial infarction. Renal blood flow is decreased, potentially resulting in renal impairment or failure. Cerebrovascular accident may result from thromboemboli or decreased cerebral perfusion. These severe complications, in addition to the initial precipitating disorder, contribute to a mortality rate in excess of 50%.

The onset of HHNC is often insidious and classically occurs in the older, non-insulin-dependent individual with diabetes who has a concomitant reduction in renal function. It is typically precipitated by some form of stress (e.g., infection, trauma, surgery) that increases the release of hormones (i.e., catecholamines, glucagon, and cortisol), which raises blood glucose levels. The combination of hypovolemia and decreased renal function ultimately results in a rapid rise in blood glucose secondary to decreased urinary excretion of glucose. The mechanism responsible for the absence of elevated ketones is not fully understood, although, it has been suggested that individuals who develop HHNC still produce enough insulin to maintain normal fat metabolism but which is insufficient for normal glucose utilization. The absence of ketoacidosis and the slow onset of vague neurologic symptoms in the older adult often result in HHNC initially being misdiagnosed as a primary neurologic disorder. See Table 20-1 for a comparison of DKA and HHNC.

Potential Fluid, Electrolyte, and Acid-Base Disturbances

1. **Fluid volume deficit** due to hyperglycemia-induced osmotic diuresis. Hypovolemia is treated with either isotonic saline (0.9% NaCl) or 0.45% saline. (See Chapter 6.)
2. **Hypokalemia** due to increased urinary losses secondary to osmotic diuresis. (See Chapter 8).
3. **Hypophosphatemia** due to increased urinary losses secondary to osmotic diuresis. Hypokalemia and hypophosphatemia are treated with a combination of IV potassium chloride and potassium phosphate. (See Chapter 10.)
4. **Hypomagnesemia** due to increased urinary losses secondary to osmotic diuresis. (See Chapter 11.)
5. **Metabolic acidosis** due to retention of lactic acid secondary to hypovolemia with tissue hypoxia. Acidosis usually

will resolve with treatment (insulin and fluids) but may be treated with IV sodium bicarbonate if severe. (See Chapter 15.)

Diabetes Insipidus (DI)

DI is caused by either a deficiency in the synthesis or release of ADH from the posterior pituitary gland (neurogenic or central DI) or a decrease in kidney responsiveness to ADH (nephrogenic DI), resulting in decreased water absorption by the renal tubules. Central DI may be idiopathic or occur as a result of cerebral tumor, trauma, or hypoperfusion and will resolve with the administration of vasopressin (see Table 20-2). In contrast, nephrogenic DI responds poorly to vasopressin and may be caused by a wide variety of medications and disorders, including electrolyte imbalance (i.e., hypokalemia or hypocalcemia).

Regardless of the cause, the individual with DI excretes large volumes of extremely dilute urine. As with diabetes mellitus, the cardinal symptoms of DI are polyuria and polydipsia. These will remain the only symptoms as long as these individuals are able to drink and satisfy their thirst, thereby maintaining fluid volume. If the person is unable to access adequate amounts of water (e.g., an infant with congenital DI or the adult who is neurologically impaired), abnormal water loss will result in rapidly decreased ECF volume and increased serum sodium and osmolality. Without treatment, severe ECF and ICF dehydration, hypotension, and shock can occur. Decreased cerebral perfusion and increased serum osmolality will produce neurologic symptoms ranging from confusion, restlessness, and irritability to seizures and coma. The severity of and prognosis for DI will vary with its cause. The onset may be sudden and dramatic with cerebral trauma, or it can be gradual, as with tumors or infiltrative disease.

Text continued on page 212.

Table 20-1 Comparison of diabetic ketoacidosis (DKA) and hyperosmolar hyperglycemic nonketotic coma (HHNC)

Criterion	DKA	HHNC
Diabetes type	Usually IDDM (type I)	Usually NIDDM (type II)
Typical age-group	Any age	Usually older than 50 yr
Signs and symptoms	Polyuria, polydipsia, polyphagia, weakness, orthostatic hypotension, lethargy, changes in LOC, fatigue, nausea, vomiting, abdominal pain	Same as DKA, but slower onset and, very commonly, neurologic symptoms
Physical assessment	Dry and flushed skin, poor skin turgor, dry mucous membranes, decreased BP, tachycardia, altered LOC (irritability, lethargy, coma), Kussmaul's respirations, fruity odor to the breath	Same as DKA, but no Kussmaul's respirations or fruity odor to the breath; instead, occurrence of tachypnea with shallow respirations
History and risk factors	Recent stressors such as surgery, trauma, infection, myocardial infarction (MI); insufficient exogenous insulin; undiagnosed type I diabetes mellitus	Undiagnosed type II diabetes mellitus; recent stressors such as surgery, trauma, pancreatitis, MI, infection; high-caloric enteral or parenteral feedings in a compromised patient; use of diabetogenic drugs (e.g., phenytoin, thiazide diuretics, thyroid preparations, mannitol, corticosteroids, sympathomimetics)

Monitoring parameters

ECG: dysrhythmias associated with hyperkalemia: peaked T waves, widened QRS complex, prolonged PR interval, flattened or absent P wave. As hyperkalemia worsens, these signs progress in the order given and may lead to asystole. Hypokalemia (K^+ <3.0 mEq/L), which may produce depressed ST segments, flat or inverted T waves, or increased ventricular dysrhythmias

ECG: evidence of hypokalemia as listed with DKA

Hemodynamic measurements: CVP>3 mm Hg below patient's baseline; PADP and PAWP>4 mm Hg below patient's baseline

Diagnostic tests

Serum glucose: 200-800 mg/dl

Serum ketones: elevated

Urine glucose: positive

Urine acetone: positive

Serum osmolality: 300-350 mOsm/L

Serum pH: <7.38

Serum sodium: <137 mEq/L initially; may be elevated with severe dehydration

Serum Hct: elevated due to osmotic diuresis with hemoconcentration

BUN: elevated >20 mg/dl

Serum creatinine: >1.5 mg/dl

800-2000 mg/dl

Normal or slightly elevated

Positive

Negative

>350 mOsm/L

Normal or mildly acidotic (pH <7.40)

Elevated, normal, or low

Elevated due to hemoconcentration

Elevated

Elevated

Continued.

Table 20-1 (continued)

Criterion	DKA	HHNC
	Serum potassium: normal or elevated >5.0 mEq/L initially and then decreased	Normal or <3.5 mEq/L
	Serum phosphorus, magnesium, chloride: decreased	Decreased
Onset	Hours to days	Hours to days; can be longer
Mortality rate	<10%	>50% due to age group and complications such as CVA, thombosis, renal failure

From Sands JK. In Swearingen PL and Keen JH: Manual of critical care: applying nursing diagnoses to adult critical illness, ed 2, St. Louis, 1991, Mosby-Year Book.

PADP=pulmonary artery diastolic pressure; PAWP=pulmonary artery wedge pressure.

Table 20-2 Vasopressin preparations

Generic Name	Trade Name	Onset	Duration	Usual Dosage	Advantages/ Disadvantages	Comments
Nasal						
Vasopressin	Pitressin	Within 1 hr	4-8 hr	5-10 U b.i.d.-t.i.d.	Action decreased by nasal congestion/ discharge or atrophy of nasal mucosa	Administer by spray, cotton pledget, or dropper; used for chronic DI management
Desmopressin acetate	DDAVP	Within 1 hr	8-20 hr	0.1-0.4 ml q.d. in 1-3 doses (10-40 μg)	See above	See above; stored in refrigerator at 4° C (39.2° F)
Lypressin	Diapid	Within 1 hr	3-8 hr	7-14 μg q.i.d.	See above	See above; stored at <40° C (100° F)

Continued.

Table 20-2 *(continued)*

Generic Name	Trade Name	Onset	Duration	Usual Dosage	Advantages/ Disadvantages	Comments
Subcutaneous Vasopressin	Pitressin	½-1 hr	2-8 hr	0.25-0.5 ml (5-10 U) q3-4h prn increased thirst or urine output		Typically used in acute care setting and for emergency management Kept refrigerated at 4° C (39.2° F)
Desmopressin acetate	DDAVP, Stimate	Within ½ hr	1½-4 hr	0.5-1 ml (2-4 µg) q.d. in 2 divided doses		
Intramuscular Vasopressin tannate in oil	Pitressin tannate in oil	Within 1-2 hr	36-48 hr	0.3-1 ml (1.5-5 U) q2-3d for increased thirst or increased urine output	Longer duration of action/ slower absorption than SC route; response cumulative over 2-3 days	Stored at 13°-18° C (55°-65° F) Shake well before withdrawing from vial; can warm solution by immersing vial in warm water

Vasopressin tannate	Pitressin tannate	½-1 hr	2-8 hr	0.25-0.5 ml (5-10 U) q3-4h for increased thirst or increased urine output	Longer duration of action, which makes IM forms more desirable for chronic management	
Intravenous						
Desmopressin acetate	DDAVP	Within ½ hr	1½-4 hr	0.5-1.0 ml (2-4 µg) q.d. in 2 divided doses	Not for home use	Keep refrigerated at 4° C (39.2° F); dilute in 10-50 ml 0.9% NaCl and infuse over 15-30 min

From Sands JK: In Swearingen PL and Keen JH: Manual of critical care: applying nursing diagnoses to adult critical illness, ed 2, St Louis, 1991, Mosby-Year Book.

Potential Fluid, Electrolyte, and Acid-Base Disturbances

1. **Fluid volume deficit** due to decreased water reabsorption by the renal tubule secondary to decreased ADH production or effectiveness. It is treated with hypotonic fluid replacement and correction of the cause. (See Chapter 6.)
2. **Hypernatremia** due to increased free water loss secondary to decreased renal reabsorption of water. Hypernatremia also is corrected by hypotonic fluid replacement. Ironically, nephrogenic DI can be treated with diuretics such as thiazide that block the kidneys' ability to excrete free water. (See Chapter 7.)

Syndrome of Inappropriate Antidiuretic Hormone (SIADH)

SIADH develops as the result of excessive levels of circulating antidiuretic hormone (ADH). The causes of SIADH fall into one of three categories: (1) excessive production or release of ADH secondary to CNS disorders, such as meningitis or increased intracranial pressure; (2) respiratory disorders, such as infections and lesions, which increase the release of ADH by an unknown mechanism; and (3) ectopic ADH secretion of malignant tumors, particularly oat cell carcinoma of the lung. In the presence of increased ADH, water that normally would be excreted in the urine is *inappropriately* reabsorbed and returned to the circulation, diluting the serum sodium and decreasing serum osmolality. ECF volume expansion increases glomerular filtration and decreases the release of aldosterone, both of which act to increase urinary excretion of sodium, further reducing the serum sodium level. As the serum sodium level decreases, an osmotic gradient is created that favors an ICF shift. Increased ICF in the brain can result in cerebral edema with altered neurologic function and ultimately death if the condition is not treated.

SIADH typically is diagnosed on the basis of laboratory findings and patient history. Classic laboratory findings include serum hyponatremia and hypoosmolality, combined with inappropriately high urine sodium and osmolality. Treatment is aimed at correcting the primary problem, limiting water intake, and administering sodium. Medications such as lithium or demeclocycline, which inhibit the action of ADH on the renal tubule, also may be used.

Potential Fluid, Electrolyte and Acid-Base Disturbances

1. **Hyponatremia** due to excessive retention of water and continued urinary loss of sodium. (See Chapter 7.)
2. **Hypervolemia** due to retention of water with cellular volume expansion. (See Chapter 6.) **Note:** ECF volume expansion usually is minimized owing to the decreased stimulus to aldosterone and increased stimulus to atrial natriuretic peptide.

Acute Adrenal Insufficiency

Adrenal insufficiency (decreased production of adrenocortical hormones) occurs as a result of either dysfunction of the adrenal glands (primary) or inadequate stimulation of the adrenal glands by the anterior pituitary gland (secondary). Conditions associated with primary adrenal insufficiency include adrenalectomy, infection, tumor invasion, autoimmune disease, enzymatic deficiencies, and adrenal atrophy secondary to chronic corticosteroid therapy. A decrease in the production of adrenocortical hormones due to a reduction in functioning adrenal tissue is also termed Addison's disease. Secondary adrenal insufficiency is associated with destruction of the pituitary gland by tumors, infarcts, trauma, surgery, or infection.

Acute adrenal insufficiency is a life-threatening condition characterized by severe fluid and electrolyte imbalances related to both mineralocorticoid and glucocorticoid deficiencies. Mineralocorticoid (aldosterone) deficiency results in large urinary losses of sodium and water with the development of hyponatremia and hypovolemia. Additionally, hyperkalemia and metabolic acidosis can develop due to decreased urinary excretion of potassium and hydrogen. Glucocorticoid (cortisol) deficiency intensifies the clinical effects of hypovolemia by causing a decrease in vascular tone and decreased vascular response to catecholamines (epinephrine and norepinephrine). Severe hypotension, shock, and eventually death will occur without adequate parenteral adreno-cortical hormone and fluid replacement. Acute crises may be pre-vented by tripling replacement hormone doses during periods of stress.

Potential Fluid, Electrolyte, and Acid-Base Disturbances

1. **Hypovolemia** due to decreased reabsorption of sodium and water by the renal tubule secondary to the lack of al-dosterone. It is treated with IV isotonic (0.9%) saline so-lution and IV hydrocortisone. (See Chapter 6.)
2. **Hyperkalemia** due to decreased secretion and excretion of potassium by the renal tubule secondary to the lack of al-dosterone. Hyperkalemia is treated with kayexalate. (See Chapter 8.)
3. **Metabolic acidosis** due to decreased secretion and excre-tion of hydrogen by the renal tubule secondary to the lack of aldosterone. Severe metabolic acidosis (HCO_3^- <10 mEq/L) may be treated with IV sodium bicarbonate. (See Chapter 15.)
4. **Hyponatremia,** which may occur in chronic primary adrenocortical insufficiency due to hypovolemia-induced release of ADH with the retention of free water. (See Chapter 7.)

Cardiac Disorders

21

Congestive Heart Failure (CHF) and Pulmonary Edema

CHF develops when the heart is unable to maintain a cardiac output sufficient to meet the metabolic needs of the tissues. Causes of CHF include coronary artery disease, hypertension, cardiomyopathy, and valvular disease. As the heart fails and the cardiac output drops, there is a reduction in effective circulating volume (ECV) with poor renal blood flow. This results in a reduction in the load of sodium and water filtered by the kidney and stimulates the release of renin. Renin causes an increase in angiotensin II, a potent vasoconstrictor that increases systemic vascular resistance and the workload of the heart (afterload). Increased angiotensin II, in turn, leads to an increase in aldosterone, with retention of sodium and water by the kidneys and an increase in vascular volume (preload). Decreased ECV also stimulates the release of antidiuretic hormone (ADH), causing further retention of water by the kidneys. Because the diseased heart is unable to circulate this increased volume, the pressure within the venous circuit increases and edema develops.

When the left heart is unable to pump the blood returning from the lungs into systemic circulation, the hydrostatic pressure within the pulmonary circulation increases. If the hydrostatic pressure exceeds the pulmonary oncotic pressure, fluid leaks into the pulmonary interstitium. This results in pulmonary edema with impairment of oxygen exchange. Right ventricular failure usually occurs secondary to left ventricular failure (the right heart must work harder as the pressure in the pulmonary vasculature increases), but may occur independently in conditions such as cor pulmonale. When the right heart fails there is a backup in the venous circuit, with congestion of blood in body organs (e.g., liver and spleen) and edema formation.

Potential Fluid, Electrolyte, and Acid-Base Disturbances

1. **Fluid volume excess,** as evidenced by peripheral and pulmonary edema, due to increased secretion of aldosterone and ADH. It is treated with diuretics and fluid and sodium restriction. Inotropic agents and vasodilators are administered to improve cardiac function. (See Chapter 6.)

2. **Hyponatremia** due to increased secretion of ADH (remember ADH affects water retention only, whereas aldosterone causes retention of both sodium and water). Hyponatremia resolves with fluid restriction and correction of the primary problem. (See Chapter 7.)

3. **Hypokalemia** due to the use of potassium-wasting diuretics (e.g., furosemide). Furosemide commonly is used in the treatment of acute pulmonary edema because of its potent and rapid diuretic action when administered IV and its direct vasodilatory effect, which reduces preload. (See Chapter 8.)

4. **Respiratory alkalosis** may occur in pulmonary edema due to hypoxia-induced hyperventilation. (See Chapter 14.)

5. **Respiratory acidosis** may develop if pulmonary edema is so severe that CO_2 retention occurs along with hypoxemia. (See Chapter 13.)

6. **Metabolic acidosis** may develop in individuals in cardiogenic shock due to increased production of lactic acid by hypoxic tissues and decreased excretion of acids by the kidney. (See Chapter 15.)

Cardiogenic Shock

Shock is a state in which blood flow to peripheral tissue is inadequate for sustaining life. Usually cardiogenic shock is caused by a massive myocardial infarction (MI) that renders 40% or more of the myocardium dysfunctional secondary to necrosis or ischemia. As a result, cardiac output is reduced and all tissues suffer from inadequate perfusion. With decreased perfusion to the heart, coronary flow is reduced, impairing cardiac function, which further decreases cardiac output.

The first stage of shock is characterized by increased sympathetic discharge as the baroreceptors at the carotid sinus and aortic arch are stimulated by the drop in blood pressure. The release of epinephrine and norepinephrine is a compensatory mechanism that increases cardiac output by increasing the heart rate and contractility of the uninjured myocardium. Vasoconstriction, a mechanism that increases blood pressure, also occurs. The second or middle stage of shock is characterized by decreased perfusion to the brain, kidneys, and heart. Lactate and pyruvic acid accumulate in the tissues, and metabolic acidosis occurs secondary to anaerobic metabolism. In the late stage of shock, which is usually irreversible, compensatory mechanisms become ineffective, and multiple organ failure occurs.

Potential Fluid, Electrolyte, and Acid-Base Disturbances

1. **Fluid volume deficit** may be present due to prior diuretic therapy with potent diuretics (e.g., furosemide). (See Chapter 6.)
2. **Fluid volume excess** may be present or develop due to stimulation of the renin-angiotensin system, resulting in retention of sodium and water. Overly aggressive fluid therapy may contribute. Volume imbalances will resolve with improved cardiac function. (See Chapter 6.)
3. **Hyponatremia** may be present secondary to an increase in the release of ADH, resulting in retention of water. (See Chapter 7.)
4. **Metabolic acidosis** occurring with accumulation of lactate and pyruvic acid in the tissues secondary to decreased tissue perfusion. Severe metabolic acidosis may require treatment with IV sodium bicarbonate. (See Chapter 15.)
5. If shock is prolonged, the individual may develop acute tubularnecrosis (ATN), which can lead to multiple fluid and electrolyte disturbances. (See Chapter 22.)

Renal
Failure

22

Because the kidneys are the primary regulators of fluid and electrolyte balance, renal failure (either acute or chronic) may lead to a myriad of disturbances in fluid and electrolyte balance. This is easy to appreciate after reviewing the normal functions of the kidneys (box below).

Acute renal failure (ARF) is a sudden loss of renal function that may or may not be accompanied by oliguria. The kidneys lose the ability to maintain biochemical homeostasis, causing retention of metabolic waste and dramatic alterations in fluid, electrolyte, and acid-base balance. Although the alteration in renal function usually is reversible, ARF is associated with an overall mortality rate of 40%-60%. However, the mortality rate varies greatly with the etiology of ARF, the patient's age, and preexisting medical problems.

The causes of ARF are classified according to etiology as prerenal, intrarenal, and postrenal (Table 22-1). A decrease in renal function secondary to decreased renal perfusion but without renal parenchymal damage is termed *prerenal failure*. Causes of prerenal failure include fluid volume deficit, shock, and decreased cardiac function. If hypoperfusion has not been prolonged, restoration of renal perfusion will restore normal renal function. A reduction in urine output that occurs because of obstruction to urine flow is termed *postrenal failure*. Conditions causing postrenal failure can include neurogenic bladder, tumors, and urethral strictures. Early detection of prerenal and postrenal failure is essential because, if prolonged, they can lead to parenchymal damage.

The most common cause of *intrarenal failure,* renal failure that develops secondary to renal parenchymal damage, is acute tubular necrosis (ATN). Although typically associated with pro-

218

Functions of the Kidney

- Regulation of water and electrolyte balance. The kidneys play an important role in the regulation of sodium ion (Na^+), potassium ion (K^+), calcium ion (Ca^{2+}), magnesium ion (Mg^{2+}), hydrogen ion (H^+), chloride ion (Cl^-), phosphate ion (PO_4^{3-}), and bicarbonate ion (HCO_3^-).
- Maintenance of acid-base balance through the excretion of H^+ and the regeneration of HCO_3^-. As each hydrogen ion is moved into the renal tubule to be excreted, a bicarbonate ion is generated and returned to the extracellular fluid (ECF).
- Excretion of metabolic wastes (i.e., urea, uric acid, creatinine, and unknown toxins).
- Excretion of foreign substances (i.e., medications, poisons, food additives).
- Production of the following:
  — *Renin:* Helps to regulate vascular volume and blood pressure through the regulation of Na^+ and water.
  — *Erythropoietin:* Released in response to a low oxygen level in the renal cells, it stimulates the production of red blood cells by the bone marrow.
  —*Active form of vitamin D:* Increases the intestinal absorption of calcium, phosphorus, and magnesium; increases bone resorption (movement out) of calcium and phosphorus; and increases the reabsorption (saving) of calcium and phosphorus by the kidney. The net result is that of helping to maintain normal calcium, phosphorus, and magnesium levels.
  —*Prostaglandins:* Primarily vasodilating substances, they affect blood flow to and within the kidney and increase kidney responsiveness to the effects of antidiuretic hormone (ADH) and aldosterone.

longed ischemia (prerenal failure) or exposure to nephrotoxins, ATN also can occur after transfusion reactions, crushing injuries, or septic abortions. The clinical course of ATN is divided into three phases: oliguric (lasting approximately 7–21 days); diuretic (lasting 7–14 days); and recovery (which can continue for 3–12

Table 22-1 Causes of acute renal failure

Prerenal (Decreased Renal Perfusion)	Intrarenal (Parenchymal Damage; Acute Tubular Necrosis)	Postrenal (Obstruction)
Fluid volume deficit	**Nephrotoxic agents**	Calculi
■ GI losses	■ Antibiotics (aminoglycosides, sulfonamides, methicillin)	**Tumor**
■ Hemorrhage	■ Diuretics (e.g., furosemide)	**Benign prostate hypertrophy**
■ Third-space (interstitial) losses (burns, peritonitis)	■ Nonsteroidal anti-inflammatory drugs (e.g., ibuprofen)	**Necrotizing papillitis**
■ Dehydration from diuretic use	■ Contrast media	Urethral strictures
Hepatorenal syndrome	■ Heavy metals (lead, gold, mercury)	**Blood clots**
Edema-forming conditions	■ Organic solvents (carbon tetrachloride, ethylene glycol)	**Retroperitoneal fibrosis**
■ Congestive heart failure	**Infection (gram-negative sepsis), pancreatis, peritonitis**	Neurogenic bladder
■ Cirrhosis		
■ Nephrotic syndrome	**Transfusion reaction (hemolysis)**	
Renal vascular disorders		
■ Renal artery stenosis		
■ Renal artery thrombosis		
■ Renal vein thrombosis		

Rhabdomyolysis with myoglobinuria (severe muscle injury)

- Trauma
- Exertion
- Seizures
- Drug-related: heroin, barbiturates, IV amphetamines, succinylcholine

Glomerular diseases

- Poststreptococcal glomerulonephritis
- IgA nephropathy (e.g., Berger's disease)
- Lupus glomerulonephritis
- Serum sickness

Ischemic injury (prolonged prerenal)

222 Clinical Conditions: Fluid, Electrolyte, Acid-Base Imbalance

months). Causes of intrarenal failure other than ATN include acute glomerulonephritis, malignant hypertension, and hepatorenal syndrome. See Table 22-2 for a list of drugs that require dosage modification for patients with ARF.

Chronic renal failure (CRF) is a progressive, irreversible loss of renal function that develops over months to years. Eventually it can progress to end-stage renal disease (ESRD), at which time renal replacement therapy (dialysis or transplantation) is required to sustain life. Prior to ESRD, the individual with CRF can lead a relatively normal life managed by diet and medications. The length of this period varies, depending on the cause of renal failure and the patient's level of renal function at the time of diagnosis.

There are many causes of CRF, some of the most common being glomerulonephritis, diabetes mellitus, hypertension, and polycystic kidney disease. Regardless of the cause, the clinical presentation of CRF, particularly as the individual approaches ESRD, is similar. Retention of nitrogenous wastes and accompanying fluid and electrolyte imbalances adversely affect all body systems. Alterations in neuromuscular, cardiovascular, and gastrointestinal function are common. Renal osteodystrophy is an early and frequent complication. These collective manifestations of CRF are termed *uremia*.

Potential Fluid, Electrolyte, and Acid-Base Disturbances

1. **Hypervolemia** due to anuria or oliguria. It is treated with fluid restriction, diuretics and, if necessary, dialysis. See Figures 22-1 and 22-2 for depictions of dialysis. (See Chapter 6.)
2. **Hypovolemia** during the diuretic phase of ARF due to excretion of large volumes of hypotonic urine, combined with existing fluid restriction. Hypovolemia also may occur in postrenal failure after release of the obstruction (post-obstructive diuresis). Hypovolemia may be the precipitating event in prerenal failure (see Table 22-1). (See Chapter 6.)
3. **Hyponatremia** due to excessive consumption or administration of hypotonic fluids. (See Chapter 7.)

Table 22-2 Drugs that require dosage modification in renal failure

Antimicrobials	Cardiovascular Agents	Analgesics	Sedatives	Miscellaneous	Drugs to Avoid
Amikacin	Digoxin	Meperidine	Phenobarbital	Insulin	Tetracycline
Gentamicin	Digitoxin	Methadone	Meprobamate	Cimetidine	Nitrofurantoin
Kanamycin	Procainamide			Clofibrate	Spironolactone
Tobramycin	Guanethidine			Neostigmine	Amiloride
Amphotericin B					Aspirin
Vancomycin					Lithium carbonate
Lincomycin					Cisplatin
Sulfonamides					Phenylbutazone
Ethambutol					Nonsteroidal anti-inflammatory agents
Penicillins					Magnesium-containing medications

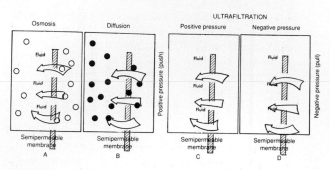

Figure 22-1.   Dialysis is based on the principles of osmosis
(**A**), diffusion (**B**), and ultrafiltration. Ultrafiltration occurs
when either positive pressure (**C**) or negative pressure (**D**) is
placed on the system. Ultrafiltration can be maximized by ex-
erting both positive and negative pressure on the system simultaneously. (From Phipps W: Medical-surgical nursing, ed
4, St Louis, 1991, Mosby-Year Book.)

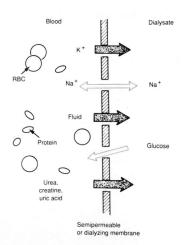

Figure 22-2.   Osmosis and diffusion in dialysis. Net movement
of major particles and fluid is illustrated. (From Phipps W:
Medical-surgical nursing, ed 4, St Louis, 1991, Mosby-Year
Book.)

4. **Hyperkalemia** due to the kidneys' inability to excrete potassium and increased tissue catabolism with the release of intracellular potassium. Hyperkalemia is managed by a combination of dietary restrictions and removal *via* cation exchange resins or dialysis. Acute, life-threatening hyperkalemia may be temporarily corrected by the administration of glucose and insulin or sodium bicarbonate. (See Chapter 8.)

5. **Hypokalemia** during the diuretic phase of ARF, especially in the potassium-restricted patient. See Chapter 8.

6. **Hyperphosphatemia** due to the kidneys' inability to excrete phosphorus. It is treated by limiting dietary intake of high phosphorus foods and administration of phosphorus-binding antacids. (See Chapter 10.)

7. **Hypocalcemia** due to decreased levels of the metabolically active form of vitamin D, hyperphosphatemia (remember that calcium and phosphorus have a reciprocal relationship: as one increases, the other tends to decrease), skeletal resistance to PTH (the hormone released by the parathyroid gland in response to a low serum calcium level), and hypoalbuminemia. Treatment begins with regulation of phosphorus *via* calcium carbonate antacids. Later Vitamin D replacement and additional calcium supplements may be necessary. (See Chapter 9.)

8. **Hypermagnesemia** due to the kidneys' inability to excrete magnesium. Hypermagnesemia usually can be prevented by avoiding magnesium-containing medications and supplements. (See Chapter 11.)

9. **Metabolic acidosis** due to the kidneys' inability to excrete the body's daily load of nonvolatile acid. Limiting dietary intake of protein and preventing tissue catabolism help to minimize acidosis. Dialysis provides some buffer replacement through the addition of bicarbonate or acetate to the dialysate. See Figures 22-1 and 22-2 for depictions of dialysis. (See Chapter 15.)

Acute Pancreatitis

23

Acute pancreatitis is a potentially life-threatening condition caused by abnormal activation of pancreatic enzymes. A variety of conditions are associated with pancreatitis, including trauma and infection; however, the most common are chronic alcoholism and biliary tract disease (see box on p. 227). Although the exact pathogenesis is unknown, injury to acinar cells results in the release and activation of pancreatic enzymes, causing autodigestion of the gland. Damage to the pancreas can range from acute edema to necrosis and hemorrhage. The individual with acute pancreatitis experiences acute abdominal pain and tenderness that may be precipitated by a meal or heavy alcohol intake. Nausea, weakness, ileus, diaphoresis, tachycardia, and hypotension often are present. Laboratory findings include elevated levels of serum amylase, serum lipase, and urine amylase and decreased levels of serum calcium and serum albumin. Inflammation and decreased vascular volume also are present.

Several potentially severe complications may accompany acute pancreatitis. The most common complication is intravascular fluid volume deficit secondary to loss of fluid into the interstitium and retroperitoneum. Release of vasoactive amines results in increased capillary permeability, vasodilatation, and depressed myocardial function. Hypoalbuminemia and hemorrhage from rupture of necrotic pancreatic vessels also may contribute to intravascular volume loss. Hypovolemia and hypotension, in turn, can lead to the development of prerenal acute renal failure (ARF) and shock. Other severe complications include tetany secondary to severe hypocalcemia, respiratory failure, and rupture of abscessed pancreatic pseudocytes.

Precipitating Factors for Acute Pancreatitis

Mechanical blockage of pancreatic ducts
- Biliary tract disease (e.g., gallstones)
- Structural abnormalities (e.g., pancreas divisum)

Toxic/metabolic factors
- Alcohol
- Hypertriglyceridemia
- Hypercalcemia (e.g., hyperparathyroidism)

Infection

Trauma
- External
- Surgical
- Iatrogenic

Ischemia
- Prolonged/severe shock
- Vasculitis

Tumors

Drugs
- Nonsteroidal antiinflammatory drugs (NSAIDs)
- Estrogens
- Corticosteroids
- Thiazides
- Tetracycline
- Sulfonamides

From Keen JH: In Swearingen PL and Keen JH: Manual of critical care:
applying nursing diagnoses to adult critical illness, ed 2, St Louis, 1991,
Mosby-Year Book.

Potential Fluid, Electrolyte, and Acid-Base Disturbances

1. **Fluid volume deficit** due to loss of fluid into the interstitium and retroperitoneum, vomiting, gastric suction, diarrhea, diaphoresis, and hemorrhage. Hypovolemia is primarily treated with crystalloids, although colloids such as albumin may be added. A large volume of parenteral fluids will be required if shock is present. No oral fluids are administered until the patient is pain free and has bowel sounds. Calcium, potassium, and magnesium are added to

IV fluids as needed (See 3, 4, and 5 below). (See Chapter 6.)

2. **Hyponatremia** may develop due to loss of sodium-rich fluids, accompanied by hypovolemia-induced increase in antidiuretic hormone (ADH) secretion. (See Chapter 7.)

3. **Hypocalcemia** due to calcium deposition in areas of fat necrosis, decreased secretion of parathyroid hormone (PTH) (remember that PTH is the primary regulator of serum calcium levels), hypoalbuminemia, and ARF (if it develops). IV calcium gluconate is indicated for the treatment of significant or symptomatic hypocalcemia. Calcium should be administered with caution as hypercalcemia has been associated with the development of pancreatitis. (See Chapter 9.)

4. **Hypomagnesemia** due to abnormal GI losses and deposition of magnesium in areas of fat necrosis. See Chapter 11.

5. **Hypokalemia** may occur due to abnormal GI losses. (See Chapter 8.)

6. **Respiratory alkalosis** may develop in the patient with respiratory complications due to hypoxemia-induced hyperventilation. (See Chapter 14.)

Hepatic Failure

24

Hepatic failure is a severe loss of liver function that may develop rapidly, as with viral or drug-induced (see box, p. 230) hepatitis, or slowly, as with Laennec's cirrhosis. In the pediatric population, it also may occur as the result of Reye's syndrome or genetic disorders. As liver insufficiency progresses, normal functions of the liver, such as nutrient, hormone, and bilirubin metabolism, are lost. Elevated bilirubin levels, combined with decreased production of bile, lead to jaundice and a deficiency of the fat-soluble vitamins A, D, and K. Lack of adequate vitamin K, combined with decreased hepatic production of several clotting factors, decreased clearance of activated clotting factors, and thrombocytopenia, result in the bleeding tendency that is common in persons with hepatic failure. Decreased synthesis of albumin, in conjunction with intrahepatic vascular obstruction, contributes to the development of ascites and decreased intravascular volume (see discussion on p. 230). Reduced vascular volume stimulates the release of renin, angiotensin, aldosterone, and antidiuretic hormone (ADH), which collectively act on the kidneys to conserve sodium and water, potentiating the development of ascites and contributing to peripheral edema.

Loss of liver function results in dysfunction in other organs, such as the brain, lungs, and kidneys. The damaged liver is unable to metabolize substances such as ammonia, which are toxic to the brain. Although the exact pathogenesis of hepatic encephalopathy remains unclear, elevated ammonia levels are associated with worsening encephalopathy. Hepatorenal syndrome, a type of acute renal failure that develops with advanced hepatic disease, is believed to develop due to unopposed renal vasoconstriction secondary to chronic release of renin, ADH, and norepinephrine. Decreased hepatic synthesis of prostaglandin precursors may limit normal renal protective mechanisms. Circulatory

Drugs with Hepatotoxic Potential

Acetaminophen	Hydrochlorothiazide
Ampicillin	Isoniazid
Carbamazepine	Ketoconazole
Carbenicillin	Methotrexate
Carbon tetrachloride	Methyldopa
Chloramphenicol	Nitrofurantoin
Chlorpromazine	Oral contraceptives
Chlorpropamide	Penicillin
Clindamycin	Phenytoin
Cocaine	Propylthiouracil
Dantrolene	Rifampin
Diazepam	Salicylates
Ethanol	Sulfonamides
Floxuridine (FUDR)	Tetracyclines (especially
(intraarterial)	parenteral)
Halothane	Verapamil

From Keen JH: In Swearingen PL and Keen JH: Manual of critical care: applying nursing diagnoses to adult critical illness, ed 2, St Louis, 1991, Mosby–Year Book.

changes also occur in the lungs with the development of a significant ventilation-perfusion mismatch. Hyperventilation and respiratory alkalosis also are common.

Potential Fluid, Electrolyte, and Acid-Base Disturbances

1. **Alterations in fluid volume** may be present as evidenced by ascites and peripheral edema. Ascites occurs in cirrhosis due to hepatic venous obstruction and retention of sodium and water by the kidney, which together increase the hydrostatic pressure in the sinusoids, favoring movement of fluid into the peritoneal space. The increased sodium and water retention that occurs with ascites is believed to be caused both by abnormal handling of sodium and water by the kidney (the overflow or overfill theory) and compensatory retention of sodium and water owing to a reduction in

effective circulating volume (ECV) that stimulates the renin-aldosterone system (the underfill theory). Reduction in ECV is the result of decreased hepatic synthesis of albumin (remember that albumin helps to hold the vascular volume in the vascular space), peripheral vasodilatation, and ascites formation itself. An increase in pressure within the peritoneal cavity caused by ascities results in increased femoral venous pressure. This, combined with hypoalbuminemia, leads to the development of peripheral edema. Edema may be treated with fluid and sodium restriction and potassium-sparing diuretics. Potassium-wasting diuretics usually are avoided due to the risk of hypokalemic alkalosis. Massive or tense ascites may require paracentesis. A peritoneovenous shunt, which drains ascitic fluid into the internal jugular vein, may be indicated for patients with refractory ascites complicated by hepatorenal syndrome. See Chapter 6 for a discussion of hypervolemia, edema, and diuretics. Note that intravascular hypovolemia may develop with excessive use of diuretics or rapid removal of ascitic fluid.

2. **Hyponatremia** is common in cirrhotic patients with ascites and edema, especially in the terminal stage. Hyponatremia is dilutional and is the result of abnormal renal handling of water. (See Chapter 7.)

3. **Hypokalemia** is commonly seen in the cirrhotic patient with ascites and edema. Causes of hypokalemia in these individuals include poor dietary intake, administration of potassium-wasting diuretics, elevated aldosterone levels (remember that aldosterone causes an increased urinary excretion of potassium), magnesium depletion (hypomagnesemia often is associated with hypokalemia), and vomiting. **Note:** Hypokalemia may cause an increase in serum ammonia levels and precipitate hepatic coma. Use of potassium-sparing diuretics helps prevent hypokalemia. (See Chapter 8.)

4. **Hyperkalemia** may occur when the liver disease is complicated by renal failure or use of potassium-sparing diuretics (see Chapter 6 for a discussion of diuretic therapy). (See Chapter 8.)

5. **Hypocalcemia** may occur in alcoholic cirrhosis due to magnesium depletion (hypomagnesemia causes a reduc-

tion in the release and action of PTH) or poor oral intake. (See Chapter 10.)

6. **Hypomagnesemia** may occur in alcoholic cirrhosis due to poor oral intake, decreased GI absorption, abnormal GI losses, and increased urinary excretion. (See Chapter 11.)

7. **Hypophosphatemia** occurs with chronic alcoholism, especially during acute withdrawal, secondary to poor dietary intake, increased GI losses with vomiting and diarrhea, use of phosphorus-binding antacids, hyperventilation (respiratory alkalosis causes an intracellular shift of phosphorus), and increased urinary losses. (See Chapter 10.)

8. **Respiratory alkalosis** may occur in all types of liver disease. The exact cause is unknown. Alkalosis increases the cellular uptake of ammonia and, combined with hypokalemia, may precipitate hepatic coma. (See Chapter 14.)

9. **Metabolic alkalosis** also may occur in the setting of liver failure owing to diuretic therapy (see Chapter 6 for a discussion of metabolic alkalosis and diuretic therapy). (See Chapter 16.)

10. **Metabolic acidosis** may develop in severe chronic liver disease due to the liver's inability to eliminate lactic acid, the presence of alcoholic- and starvation-induced ketoacidosis, renal failure with the retention of acids, and the loss of bicarbonate in diarrhea. (See Chapter 15.)

Burns

25

The skin is a complex organ that provides the body's first line of defense against a potentially hostile environment. It protects against infection, prevents loss of body fluids, helps control body temperature, functions as an excretory and sensory organ, aids in activating vitamin D, and influences body image. Burns are a common, yet largely preventable form of skin injury. In the initial phase of thermal injury, marked shifts in fluids and electrolytes pose the greatest risk to recovery. The immediate goal of therapy for major burns is preservation of vital organ function in the presence of significant hypovolemia and acidosis. The challenge of treatment is to maintain vascular volume and tissue perfusion with a minimum of edema formation.

In burns covering less than 30% of the body, fluid shifts are limited to the area of burn injury. Injured tissues release chemical mediators that increase local capillary permeability, allowing both colloids and crystalloids to move into the interstitial space. Increased capillary permeability is greatest during the first 8–12 hours postburn, although full recovery of capillary integrity does not occur for 2–3 days. When burns cover more than 30% of the body, fluid shifts occur in both burned and nonburned tissue. The edema that develops in nonburned tissue is believed to be caused largely by hypoproteinemia resulting from loss of protein into burned tissue and to a lesser extent by the action of circulating vasoactive substances. In addition, thermal injury decreases cell membrane potential, allowing sodium and water to enter the cells, causing cellular swelling. The loss of skin also leads to a direct loss of fluid and heat from the body. Metabolic acidosis develops due to decreased tissue perfusion. Inhalation injury or injury to the upper airways with development of tissue edema limits the ability of the lungs to compensate for acidosis *via* hyperventilation. Severe inhalation injury may lead to profound hypoxemia and respiratory acidosis that require mechanical ventilation.

Burns are classified according to wound depth and are described either as partial- or full-thickness burns, depending on the layer of skin involved. Partial-thickness burns, which involve the epidermis, may be either superficial, i.e., dry, without blisters and edema or deep, i.e., moist, with blisters, blebs, and edema and involving the epidermis and varying levels of the dermis. Full-thickness burns destroy all epidermal elements and require skin grafting if they are larger than 4 cm in diameter. See Table 25-1 for characteristics of the various types of burns.

One of the first steps in burn therapy is to determine the extent of the burn wound (see Figures 25-1 and 25-2) and magnitude of the burn injury (Table 25-2). Burn magnitude and severity will determine whether the patient requires transfer to a specialized burn center for treatment. See Table 25-3 for factors that determine burn severity. Knowledge of the extent of the burn wound is essential in estimating the volume of fluid needed to replace that which is lost into the tissues.

Aggressive fluid replacement is necessary during the initial resuscitation phase. Several formulas advocating the use of both crystalloids and colloids have been developed to direct fluid therapy (Table 25-4). Some formulas recommend crystalloids for the first 24 hours with a switch primarily to colloids on the second day. Others recommend the use of both crystalloids and colloids during the first 24 hours postburn. In either case, the key to effective treatment is the tailoring of fluid therapy to the individual's need and response to fluid replacement.

Mobilization of edema begins at approximately 72 hours postburn. Intravascular fluid overload with congestive heart failure is a risk at this time. Because the body must rid itself of excess fluid that was required during the initial acute phase, massive diuresis of fluid is expected, and this loss should not be replaced fully. Careful monitoring of hemodynamic status is essential during this phase to prevent dangerous fluid volume changes.

Potential Fluid, Electrolyte, and Acid-Base Disturbances

1. **Hypovolemia** due to increased capillary permeability, with loss of intravascular fluid and proteins into the inter-

Table 25-1   Characteristics of burn wound depth

	Partial-Thickness	Full-Thickness
Cause	Flash, flame, ultraviolet (sunburn), hot liquid or solid, chemicals, radiation	Flame, hot liquid or solid, chemical, electrical, radiation
Surface appearance	*Superficial:* Dry, no blisters or edema *Deep:* Moist blebs, blisters, edema, oozing of plasma-like fluid.	Dry, leathery, eschar. Thrombosed blood vessels may be visible.
Color	Cherry red to mottled white; will blanch and refill.	Ranges in color from red to khaki-colored; waxy; charred; does not blanch.
Sensation	*Superficial:* Very painful to the touch. *Deep:* Extremely sensitive to touch, temperature, and air currents.	Anesthetic to touch and temperature because of destruction of sensory nerve endings.
Healing	3-35 days.	Wounds ≥4 cm must be grafted.

From Kresge E. In Swearingen PL and Keen JH: Manual of critical care, ed 2, St. Louis, 1991, Mosby–Year Book.

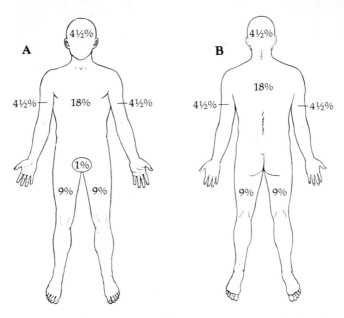

Figure 25-1.   Estimation of adult burn injury: rule of nines. **A,** Anterior view; **B,** Posterior view. From Thompson JM et al: Mosby's manual of clinical nursing, 2nd ed. St Louis: 1989, Mosby—Year Book.

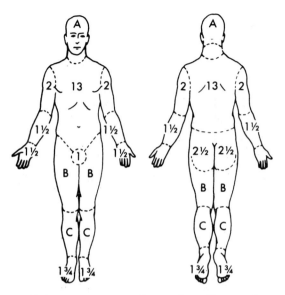

Relative percentages of areas affected by growth
(age in years)

	0	1	5	10	15	Adult
A: half of head	9½	8½	6½	5½	4½	3½
B: half of thigh	2¾	3¼	4	4¼	4½	4¾
C: half of leg	2½	2½	2¾	3	3¼	3½

Second degree _____ and

Third degree _____ =

Total percent burned——

Figure 25-2. Estimation of burn injury: Lund and Browder chart. Areas designated by letters (**A, B,** and **C,**) represent percentages of body surface area that vary according to age. The accompanying table indicates the relative percentages of these areas at various stages in life.

Table 25-2 ABA classification system

| Magnitude of Burn Injury | Second-Degree | | Third-Degree: Adults and Children % BSA | Special Location* | Complications, Poor Risk, Fractures, Other Trauma |
	Adult % BSA	Children % BSA			
Major	>25%	>20%	>10%	+	+
Moderate	15-25%	10-20%	<10%	−	−
Minor	<15%	<10%	<2%	−	−

*Special location: Hands, face, eyes, feet, and/or genitalia.

BSA = body surface area.

From Kresge E. In Swearingen PL and Keen JH: Manual of critical care, ed 2, St. Louis, 1991, Mosby–Year Book.

Table 25-3   Factors determining burn severity

Extent	Severity dependent on intensity and duration of exposure.
Depth	Severity dependent on intensity and duration of exposure.
Age	Patients <2 years old and >60 years of age.
Medical History	Preexisting conditions such as heart disease, chronic renal failure.
Body part	Special burn areas: hands, face, eyes, ears, feet, and genitalia.
Complications	Burns with concomitant trauma (i.e., fractures).

From Kresge E. In Swearingen PL and Keen JH: Manual of critical care, ed 2, St. Louis, 1991, Mosby–Year Book.

stitium, and evaporative loss of fluid through the burn wound. The plasma-to-interstitial fluid shift occurs during the first 2-3 days. Later, there is a shift of fluid from the interstitium back into the plasma. **Hypervolemia** may develop at this time, especially if there has been aggressive fluid replacement during the initial phase. As discussed, fluid replacement may involve the use of both crystalloids (usually lactated Ringer's solution) and colloids (usually albumin). Hypertonic sodium chloride solutions have been advocated by some burn centers. (See Chapter 6.)

2. **Hyponatremia** due to hypovolemia-induced increase in ADH. Sodium chloride is administered to maintain the serum sodium level within an acceptable range. (See Chapter 7.)

3. **Hyperkalemia** due to release of potassium from damaged cells. This is most likely to occur when the burn injury is complicated by acute renal failure. **Hypokalemia** may develop during the recovery phase due to shift of potassium back into the cells and increased excretion of potassium in the urine. (See Chapter 8.)

4. **Hypocalcemia** may develop due to loss of extracellular fluid from the burn wound and shift of calcium to the wound. (See Chapter 9.)

Table 25-4 Formulas for fluid replacement resuscitation

Formulas	First 24 Hours		
	Electrolyte	Colloid	Glucose in Water
ABA Consensus	Lactated Ringer's solution, 2-4 ml/kg/% BSA to maintain urinary output at 30-50 ml/hr		
Brooke	Lactated Ringer's solution, 1.5 ml/kg/% burn	0.5 ml/kg/% burn	2000 ml
Parkland	Lactated Ringer's solution, 4 ml/kg/% burn		
Hypertonic sodium solution	Volume to maintain urinary output at 30 ml/hr (fluid contains 250 mEq sodium/L)		

BSA = body surface area.
From Thelan LA, Davie JK: Textbook of critical care nursing. St Louis: 1990, Mosby–Year Book.

5. **Hypophosphatemia** commonly is associated with burns and occurs several days after the burn injury. The exact cause is unknown, but it may occur due to elevated calcitonin levels or respiratory alkalosis. (See Chapter 10.)

6. **Metabolic acidosis** may occur due to release of acids from damaged tissue and production of lactic acid if hypovolemia has led to shock. Metabolic acidosis can be avoided or

Second 24 Hours		
Electrolyte	Colloid	Glucose in Water
One half to three quarters of first 24-hr requirement	One half to three quarters of first 24-hr requirement	2000 ml
	20%-60% of calculated plasma volume	
One third of salt solution orally, up to 3500 ml limit		

minimized by early treatment of fluid volume deficit. (See Chapter 15.)

7. **Respiratory alkalosis** may develop due to hyperventilation secondary to pain and anxiety. (See Chapter 14).

8. **Respiratory acidosis** may develop with severe inhalation injury. (See Chapter 13.)

Providing Nutritional Support

26

The primary goal of nutritional support is to meet the patient's needs for maintenance of core body temperature, metabolic processes, and tissue repair. Reports indicate that approximately 50% of selected surgical patients have demonstrated signs of protein-calorie malnutrition (Lowry, 1989); however, the ability to predict increased mortality and morbidity because of malnutrition remains uncertain.

Nutritional Assessment

The need for nutritional support is based on the following components, and on patient history and history of the disease process.

Nutrition Data Collection

1. **Dietary history:** Taken to reveal the adequacy of usual and recent food intake. In addition to noting excesses or deficiencies of nutrients, determine special eating patterns (e.g., various types of vegetarian or prescribed diets), use of fad diets, or excessive supplementation. Of particular concern is anything that impairs adequate selection, preparation, ingestion, digestion, absorption, and excretion of nutrients. Include the following:
   - Comprehensive review of usual dietary intake, including food allergies, food aversions, and use of nutritional supplements.
   - Recent unplanned weight gain or loss.
   - Chewing or swallowing difficulties.
   - Nausea, vomiting, or pain with eating.

- Diarrhea, constipation, or any alteration in the pattern of elimination.
- Chronic disease affecting utilization of nutrients, e.g., malabsorption, pancreatitis, diabetes mellitus.
- Surgical resection or disease of the gut or accessory organs of digestion (pancreas, liver, gallbladder).
- Use of alcohol or drugs. Be sure to note chronic use of drugs that affect appetite, digestion, or the utilization or excretion of nutrients.

2. **Physical examination:** An adequate physical examination to determine nutritional status should include assessment for the following:
   - Loss of muscle and adipose tissue.
   - Organ dysfunction.
   - Changes in skin, hair, or neuromuscular function.

3. **Anthropomorphic data:** Measurement of the body or its parts. Because of the potential for inaccuracy in measurement, a diagnosis of malnutrition should be based on at least three abnormal parameters. It is helpful to remember that 1 L of fluid equals approximately 2 1b. Pounds and inches are converted to metric measurements using the following formulas:

   divide pounds by 2.2 to convert to kilograms

   divide inches by 39.37 to convert to meters

   - *Height:* Used to determine ideal weight and body mass index.
     —Obtain estimate from family or significant others.
     —Patient's recumbent length may be compared with known length of mattress.
   - *Weight:* One of the most readily available and practical indicators of adequacy of nutritional status.
     —Compare with ideal body weight or use to calculate body mass index.
     —Changes may reflect fluid shifts (edema, diuresis, third spacing); surgical resection; traumatic amputations; or weight of dressings or equipment.
   - *Body mass index (BMI):* Used to evaluate adult weight. One calculation and set of standards is applicable for both men and women.

$$\text{BMI (kg/m}^2) = \frac{\text{Weight (kg)}}{\text{Height (meters)} \times \text{Height (meters)}}$$

BMI values of 20–25 are optimum; values >25 indicate obesity; values <20 indicate underweight status.

- *Triceps skin fold thickness and arm circumference:* Because of the variation among evaluators, changes are difficult to identify and hence inaccurate to use as a basis for a diagnosis of malnutrition.

4. **Biochemical data:**
   - *Albumin:* With a relatively long half-life of 20 days, albumin is a less sensitive index of current nutritional status, although it remains a critical nutritional marker. Normal range is 3.5–5.5 g/dl.
   - *Transferrin:* With a half-life of 8 days, this globulin protein to which iron is bound, is a powerful indicator (in the absence of anemia) of current nutritional status. In the presence of iron deficiency anemia there is an increase in transferrin concentration, which decreases its sensitivity as a nutritional marker. Normal range is 250–420 mg/dl.
   - *Prealbumin:* With a half-life of 2 days, it correlates closely with transferrin levels and nitrogen balance and is a sensitive marker of nutritional status. Its use may be affected by its cost and availability. Normal range is 10–40 mg/dl.
   - *Delayed cutaneous hypersensitivity (DCH):* Measures the degree of responsiveness by a patient to a series of antigens. A well-nourished individual will have a positive skin reaction, whereas one who is not will have little or no reaction. Although a lack of reaction often is caused by malnutrition, in the critically ill its lack of specificity makes it less sensitive in assessing nutrition. Further, it takes longer to perform and is more expensive than other tests.

5. **Ultrasonography:** Technique for differentiating and measuring body fat and lean muscle. It is suggested that it is a more accurate indicator of nutritional status than anthropometry, and further research will determine its usefulness.

Estimating Energy Requirements

Having collected all data, energy needs can now be estimated using the following options.

1. **Indirect calorimetry:** Performed using a bedside metabolic cart. Specialized personnel are required to provide accurate results.
2. **Estimation based on Harris & Benedict equations of basal energy expenditure (BEE):** W = weight in kg; H = height in cm; A = age in years.

BEE (male) = 66.5 + (13.8 × W) + (5 × H) − (6.8 × A).

BEE (female) = 655.1 + (9.6 × W) + (1.9 × H) − (4.7 × A).

Having calculated resting energy expenditure, the appropriate correction factors, suggested by Long and co-workers (1979), should be applied to allow for the patient's activity level and condition:

Activity factor = 1.2 for bedridden patient
                  1.3 for ambulatory patient
Injury factor = 1.2 for minor surgery
                1.35 for trauma (blunt or skeletal)
                1.6 for major sepsis
                2.1 for severe burns

BEE × activity factor × injury factor = TEE (total energy expenditure).

3. **Monitoring of 24-hour urine specimens:** To ascertain nitrogen excretion, which is proportional to BEE, and electrolyte needs. A patient's protein and electrolyte needs, which change depending on the stage of illness, can be more closely approximated by monitoring the excretion rates of urea, creatinine, sodium, and potassium.
4. **Nitrogen balance:** A positive nitrogen balance is present when nitrogen intake is greater than its excretion and an anabolic state exists. If more nitrogen is excreted than taken in, nitrogen balance is said to be negative and a catabolic state exists. Most nitrogen loss occurs through the urine, with a small, constant amount lost *via* the skin and

feces. Nitrogen balance studies should be performed by specialists. Accurate measurement of 24-hour food intake and urine output is required. During critical illness, the goal is nitrogen balance, which provides sufficient protein for wound repair and other metabolic functions. A positive nitrogen state in critical illness may be deleterious because it stimulates liver function and carbon dioxide production.

5. **Distribution of calories:** As a general guide, the percentages of total calories from protein, carbohydrates, and fat should equal 15%, 50%, and 35%, respectively. Nonprotein calorie requirements are 1.2 to 1.5 times BEE in enteral nutrition and 1.5 to 2.0 times BEE during parenteral nutrition.

- *Protein requirements:* Unlike simple starvation, surgery, trauma, and sepsis alter the usual pattern of nutrient utilization. Body protein, not fat, becomes the fuel of choice. Protein requirements in critical illness usually are 1-1.5 g/kg/day.

- *Carbohydrate requirements:* Glucose administration of 5 mg/kg/min is a suitable amount. Carbohydrates provided in excess are not well utilized and may lead to hyperglycemia, excessive CO_2 production, hypophosphatemia, and fluid overload.

- *Fat requirements:* If protein and glucose are supplied as outlined, providing the remainder of needed calories as fat will meet overall needs. Fat can be administered in minimal quantities to satisfy needs for essential fatty acids, or it can be provided in larger quantities, as tolerated, to meet energy needs, especially in the patient being weaned from ventilator support with CO_2 retention as a complicator. Abnormal liver function often occurs in patients maintained on total parenteral nutrition (TPN) for more than 3 weeks. Usually the enzymes return to normal upon cessation of TPN. Giving cyclic TPN, in which the patient receives TPN for 12–16 hours out of 24 hours, sometimes helps.

- *Special formulated diets:* Requirements and limitations created by organ-specific pathology are met by the following:

—*Hepatic failure:* Branched-chain amino acids in combination with reduced aromatic amino acid concentrations are used to alleviate encephalopathy secondary to hepatocellular dysfunction.

—*Renal failure:* Intact or keto analogs of essential amino acids are used to improve nitrogen untilization in acute renal failure.

—*Respiratory failure:* A low-protein and low-carbohydrate diet decreases minute ventilation and consequently the work of breathing, which makes weaning from mechanical ventilation easier.

—*Sepsis, trauma:* Branched chain amino acids are used to achieve positive nitrogen balance. Controversy remains over the respective merits of a diet high in carbohydrates or fats in patients who are highly stressed.

6. **Fluid requirements:** Many factors affect fluid balance. Under usual circumstances an estimate of fluid needs can be made by providing 1 ml of free water for each calorie provided or 30 to 50 ml/kg/body weight. All sources of intake (oral, enteral, intravenous, and medications) as well as output (urine, stool, drains, fistulae, emesis, fluid shifts, and expiratory and evaporative losses) must be taken into consideration.

7. **Vitamins and essential trace mineral requirements:**

   ▪ In general, follow the recommended daily allowance (RDA) to provide at least minimum quantities of vitamins, minerals, and essential fatty acid supplementation.

   ▪ For specific patients, supplement vitamins or minerals known to be needed in increased amounts for existing disease states (e.g., zinc and vitamins A and C for burns; thiamine, folate, and vitamin B_{12} for chronic alcohol ingestion).

Nutritional Support Modalities

Enteral Nutrition

Enteral nutrition is that which is provided *via* the gastrointestinal tract. Oral enteral nutrition is taken by mouth; tube enteral nutrition is provided through a tube or catheter that delivers nutrients distal to the oral cavity.

Enteral Products

Products for normal gut function range from blenderized meal "hydrolysate" (usually well tolerated) to products of variable degrees of complexity, to predigested modular diets in which the protein, fat, and carbohydrates are individually mixed (Table 26-1).

Practicalities of Enteral Feeding

1. **Definitions**
   - *Small-bore feeding tube:* Polyurethane or silicone; flexible with tunsten tip; 6–12Fr; length 36–45 inches. Trade names are Keofeed, Dobhoff.
   - *Large-bore feeding tube:* Rubber or polyvinyl chloride; 10–18 Fr; used for highly viscous fluids. Trade names are Levine, Salem.
   - *Gastric feeding tube:* Tube that is placed through the naris (nasogastric) or mouth (orogastric) into the stomach for feeding purposes.
   - *Nasointestinal feeding tube:* Tube that is placed through the naris into the intestine for feeding purposes.
   - *Gastrostomy tube:* Inserted directly into the stomach either temporarily or permanently for feeding purposes. A *gastrostomy button* has been shown to decrease many of the disadvantages of gastrostomy tubes, such as site problems, leakage, mobility, and catheter occlusion and expulsion.
   - *Jejunostomy tube:* Used for long-term nutritional support in specific patient populations (e.g., traumatic brain injury); may be permanent or temporary. Needle catheter jejunostomy is an alternative method of nutrient delivery.
2. **Selection of feeding sites**
   - *Stomach:* Patients who are alert with intact gag and cough reflexes may receive feedings intragastrically. This is the site best for hyperosmolar feedings and constant infusions. Keep the patient's head of bed elevated to 30 degrees or the bed in reverse Trendelenburg position.

— Passage of food through the pylorus depends on the ability of the stomach to secrete enzymes until the stomach contents are iso-osmotic. If a bolus of hyperosmolar fluid is administered, gastric motility decreases until gastric secretions ensure the contents are iso-osmotic, thus enabling passage through the pylorus.

— Acidic secretions, which prevent bacterial contamination of the gut, may be neutralized by continuous infusion, allowing an overgrowth of bacteria if feedings are contaminated.

- *Small bowel:* Patients who are less alert with diminished protective pharyngeal reflexes should be fed *via* a tube inserted into the duodenum (gastrostomy tube or needle catheter jejunostomy).

  — Less able to dilute osmotic loads.

  — Within the first 120 cm of jejunum, the dipeptide form of protein is more easily absorbed.

  — Carbohydrates are absorbed high in the jejunum. Simple sugars are preferred because complex sugars require enzymatic activity.

  — Fat is absorbed in the duodenum and jejunum. The process requires proper mixing with bile and release of pancreatic enzymes.

  — Intestinal cells that produce lactase and are located in the microvilli are commonly damaged in the seriously ill patient, resulting in lactase deficiency. These patients will have diarrhea when given lactose-containing products.

  — Normal functions of the gut can be severely damaged by atrophy and injury of the intestinal mucosa, resulting in translocation of bacteria. Early enteral feeding following trauma can prevent atrophy of the mucosa and decrease complications (Alexander, 1990).

3. **Infusion rates:** Controversy exists regarding whether to manipulate volume or strength and concentration (i.e., initially dilute with water, [e.g., half strength]). As a general rule, follow these guidelines:

- *Gastric:* First increase osmolality (strength or concentration), then volume.

Table 26-1   Types of enteral formulations

Enteral Formula	Description
Blenderized diet	
Compleat, Compleat Modified, Vitaneed	Nutritionally complete, requiring complete digestive capabilities; composed of natural foods including meat, vegetables, milk, and fruit.
Milk-based formula	
Meritene, Sustagen, Carnation Instant (if mixed with milk)	Nutritionally adequate diet for general nutritional support.
Lactose-free formula	
Ensure, Entrition 1, Isocal, Osmolite	Nutritionally adequate, liquid preparation; used for general nutritional support; iso- or hypo-osmolar; all except Osmolite are low residue.
Elemental or chemically defined	
Criticare	Nutrients tailored for specific needs.
Travasorb HN	Low sodium, lactose free, high nitrogen diet. 40% protein supplied as small peptides; nutritionally adequate; used for general nutritional support.
Vital HN	Nutritionally adequate; used for general nutritional support; contains additional hydrolyzed protein that is readily digested and absorbed.
	For use in hypermetabolic states; nutritionally adequate; low osmolality; low residue; low electrolyte levels; additional nitrogen from partially hydrolized proteins.

Specialty formulas

Hepatic failure

Hepatic Travasorb — Nutritionally complete with a greater ratio of branched chain to aromatic amino acids while restricting total amino acid concentrations and adding nonprotein calories.

Hepatic-Aid II — Nutritionally incomplete powder diet with essential nutrients in easily digestible form; high in branched-chain amino acids; low in aromatic amino acids and methionines.

Renal failure

Renal Travasorb — Electrolyte, lactose, fat-soluble vitamin free; high in calories; contains mostly essential amino acids; restricted total protein content may reduce or postpone the need for dialysis.

Amin-Aid — Nutritionally incomplete powder dietary supplemental containing essential nutrients in readily digestible form with minimal electrolytes.

Respiratory insufficiency

Pulmocare — A nutritionally complete product that contains a higher proportion of fat to carbohydrates; reduces CO_2 production.

Hypermetabolic and trauma states

Trauma-Aid HB — High in branched-chain amino acids; readily digestible essential nutrients.

Trauma Cal — Nutritionally adequate with high proportions of protein and calories in a limited volume.

Modular formulas — Offer highly flexible tailoring of nutrients (e.g., fat [Lipomul], protein [Pro Mod], and carbohydrates [Moducal] for specific patient needs.

Table 26-2   Methods and rates of administration for enteral products

Type	Description	Comments
Bolus	E.g., 250–400 ml 4–6/day over a few min	May cause cramping, bloating, nausea, diarrhea, aspiration
Intermittent	E.g., 250–400 mg 4–6/day over 30–60 min	Should not exceed 30 ml/min; may cause cramping, bloating, nausea, diarrhea, aspiration
Continuous	E.g., 100 ml/hr for 16–24 hr	Allows more time for absorption of nutrients

Modified from Roberts PM and Webber KS: Providing nutritional support. In Swearingen PL and Keen JH: Manual of critical care: applying nursing diagnoses to adult critical disorders, ed 2, St Louis, Mosby–Year Book, 1991.

- *Small bowel:* First increase volume, then osmolality. (See Tables 26-2 and 26-3.)
4. **Management of metabolic and other complications:** See Table 26-4.

Total Parenteral Nutrition (TPN)

Parenteral nutrition provides some or all nutrients by a means other than the gastrointestinal tract, usually intravenous. Although it is usually considered more efficacious than enteral nutrition, there is a potential increase in cardiac output when the gut is bypassed, and an increase in complications with the use of central venous access. Peripheral or central venous access can be used to supplement limited oral intake or completely meet nutritional needs.

1. **Peripheral access:** Delivered through a peripheral vein, usually of the hand or forearm, and reserved for patients with the need for nutritional support for short periods of time, small nutritional requirements, and for whom central venous access is unavailable. The types of solutions are
Text continues on page 257.

Table 26-3 Nursing implications for use of gastric tubes

Size	Nursing Implications
Small bore	Ensure that x-ray confirms placement. Auscultation is not a reliable method of determining placement; aspiration of stomach contents through the tube often causes tube walls to collapse. Tubes are easily dislocated upward in the gastrointestinal tract, although there may be no external signs and the tube still may be taped in position. Use predigested formula to lower viscosity. Flush after each feeding with 50–150 ml water. Do not use syringe smaller than 50 ml to irrigate tube because high pressures generated by smaller syringes may rupture the tube.
Large bore	Use smallest bore tube possible to minimize chance of ulceration, pharyngitis, and fistula formation. Aspirate stomach contents, and check pH of returns to ensure correct stomach placement. Stomach contents have a pH < 7 (acidic). When taping tube, ensure that there is no traction applied to patient's skin. Flush after each feeding with 50–150 ml water.

Modified from Roberts PM and Webber KS: Providing nutritional support. In Swearingen PL and Keen JH: Manual of critical care: applying nursing diagnoses to adult critical disorders, ed 2, St Louis, Mosby–Year Book, 1991.

Table 26-4 Management of complications in the tube-fed patient

Complication/Possible Causes	Suggested Management Strategy
Diarrhea	
Bolus feeding	Try intermittent or continuous method.
Infusion rate	Decrease rate of delivery.
Lactose intolerance	As prescribed, switch to lactose-free products.
Fat intolerance	Reduce fat intake during acute illness.
Osmolality intolerance	Dilute feeding or use product with lower osmolality as prescribed.
Low-fiber content	Try bulk-forming agents or fiber preparations.
Medications	Monitor use of antibiotics, antacids, antiarrhythmics, aminophylline, cimetidine, and potassium chloride. Monitor use of sorbitol in liquid medications. As prescribed, administer *Lactobacillus acidophilus* to restore gastrointestinal flora. Use tincture of opium, as prescribed, to decrease GI motility. Monitor occurrence of superinfections.
Bacterial contamination	Discard feedings hanging for >8 hr. Use clean technique; change equipment q24h; refrigerate all opened products but discard after 24 hrs.
Low serum albumin	Monitor serum albumin levels; low levels contribute to intestinal malabsorption. Normal range is 3.5–5.5 g/dl.
High gastric residual	
Decreased motility	Hold feeding for 1 hr and check residual; repeat q1–2h until feeding can be resumed. After feeding, have patient lie in a right side-lying position with HOB elevated 30 degrees. As prescribed, administer metoclopramide HCl to help prevent or treat nausea and vomiting caused by slow gastric emptying.

Nausea and vomiting

Fast rate	Decrease rate
Fat intolerance	Fat should compose no more than 30%–40% of total intake.
Lactose intolerance	As prescribed, change to lactose-free product.
Hyperosmolality	Dilute feeding.
Delayed gastric emptying	Feed beyond the pylorus *via* nasoduodenal or jejunostomy tube. As prescribed, give metoclopramide to treat or prevent nausea and vomiting. *Small bore tubes*: Auscultate for bowel sounds; percuss the abdomen for air to help determine cause.
Product odor	Mask with flavoring.

Aspiration

Head of bed too low	Raise HOB 30 degrees during and 45–60 min after feeding. Monitor breath sounds and VS and observe pulmonary secretions for blue food coloring, which has been added to feeding. Test pulmonary secretions for glucose, which reflects the presence of formula (may be falsely positive when blood is in respiratory secretions). Monitor for fever, unexplained infiltrates, and increased respiratory rate and effort, inasmuch as aspiration can occur silently and quickly.
Deflated endotracheal tube cuff	Keep cuff inflated during feeding.
Delayed gastric emptying	Feed beyond the pylorus *via* nasoduodenal or jejunostomy tube.
Incorrect tube position	*Small-bore tube*: Check x-ray for position. *Large-bore tube*: Aspirate and test stomach contents for acidity before bolus feeding and q4h for continuous feeding.

Continued.

Table 26-4 *(continued)*

Complication/Possible Causes	Suggested Management Strategy
Bolus feedings	Switch to intermittent or continuous feeding.
Blocked tube	
Inadequate flushing	Flush tube with 50–150 ml water after each feeding. Institute routine flushing with Coca Cola or water. Flush blocked tubes with proteolytic enzyme papain (Adolph's Meat Tenderizer), pancreatic enzyme (Viokase), Pepsi Cola, Mountain Dew, or cranberry juice (Nicholson, 1987; Marcuard et al 1990). The high acidity of cranberry juice and Coca Cola and the carbonation of Coca Cola, in particular, have been suggested as the reasons for their effectiveness. A device called Intro-Reducer has been designed to clear blocked soft feeding tubes.
Instillation of crushed medications	Substitute liquid preparations after consulting with pharmacist and attending MD.

Modified from Roberts PM and Webber KS: Providing nutritional support. In Swearingen PL and Keen JH: Manual of critical care: applying nursing diagnoses to adult critical disorders, ed 2, St Louis, Mosby–Year Book, 1991.

limited to those which, when infused together, have a final osmolality of < 800 mOsm/L, such as:

- 5%–10% dextrose
- 3%–5% amino acid
- 10%–20% lipid emulsion, which provides the bulk of calories

3. **Central venous access:** Used for patients who are unable to meet their nutritional needs *via* peripheral route. Solutions infused *via* central catheters usually include those which, when infused together, have a final osmolality of > 800 mOsm/L, such as:

- *Dextrose 25% to 50% (hypertonic)*
- *Amino acid formulations:* 4.25% and 5%.
- *Special amino acid formulations:* Used for patients with specific pathologies, such as:
  —*Renal failure:* Contain only essential amino acids.
  —*Hepatic encephalopathy:* Fortified with branched chain amino acids, which do not depend on liver function for metabolism.
  —*Trauma, sepsis, or highly stressed:* Fortified with branched chain amino acids.
- *Fat emulsions:* 10% to 20%
  —To enhance tolerance, fat emulsions should be infused over no fewer than 8 hours. The most common symptoms of an adverse reaction include febrile response, chills and shivering, and pain in the chest and back. A second type of adverse reaction, which occurs with prolonged use of IV fat emulsions, may result in transient increase in liver enzymes, kernicterus, eosinophilia, and thrombophlebitis.
  —Keep the infusion rate 1 ml/min for the first 15–30 min and then increase it to 80–100 ml/hr for the remainder of the first infusion.
  —To prevent sepsis, fat emulsions should hang no longer than 12 hours.
- *Total nutrient admixtures:* Relatively new type of solution in which dextrose, fat, and amino acids are combined in one container. Because it would trap lipid molecules, an in-line filter cannot be used.

Types of Catheters

1. **Single lumen:** Multiple uses for specimen retrieval, feeding, and medication administration increases the risk of infection, especially in compromised patients.
2. **Multi-lumen:** Restriction of one lumen in a multi-lumen catheter for TPN is a common practice, leaving other lumen(s) for medication administration and laboratory monitoring.
3. **Right atrial catheter:** Long-term venous access catheter.
4. **Implantable catheter:** Implanted catheter for venous and arterial access, which negates the need for repeated venipunctures; can be used for drugs, TPN, and blood products.

Monitoring Infusion Rates

An infusion pump is recommended to avoid wide fluctuations in blood glucose. For the same reason, TPN solutions should never be accelerated to "catch up," nor discontinued suddenly.

Potential Fluid, Electrolyte, and Acid-Base Disturbances

Fluid Imbalances

1. **Hypervolemia** due to overfeeding (excess volume of TPN or enteral formula) or overhydration. (See Chapter 6.)
2. **Hypovolemia** due to diarrhea, emesis, febrile states, hyperglycemia, hyperosmolar hyperglycemic nonketotic coma, and the refeeding syndrome, which causes diuresis as a result of the mobilization of edemic fluid. The latter occurs shortly after initiation of TPN in a malnourished patient who is hypoproteinemic and edematous. (See Chapters 6 and 20.)

Sodium Imbalances

1. **Hypernatremia** due to excessive sodium intake from an enteral or parenteral formula in combination with inadequate fluid intake. (See Chapter 7.)
2. **Hyponatremia** due to water overload (see Chapter 6) or inadequate sodium intake (see Chapter 7).

Table 26-5   Management of complications in the patient receiving parenteral nutrition

Potential Complications	Management Strategy
Pneumothorax	Use Trendelenburg position when catheter is inserted into central vein; check x-ray immediately after insertion. Usually small leaks resolve spontaneously.
Subclavian artery injury	If pulsative, bright red blood returns into the syringe, assist MD with immediate removal of the needle and apply pressure for 10 min anteriorly and posteriorly to the clavicle at the point of penetration.
Air embolism	Use Trendelenburg position when catheter is inserted into central vein; have patient perform Valsalva's maneuver during tubing changes. With patient receiving ventilation, change tubing during expiration phase. Tape all tubing connections longitudinally to prevent disconnection; use occlusive dressing over insertion site for 24 hrs after catheter has been removed to prevent air entry *via* catheter-sinus tract. If air embolism is suspected, place patient in left side-lying decubitus and Trendelenburg position to trap air in the right ventricle; give oxygen and CPR as necessary; contact MD stat.
Vein thrombosis	As prescribed, a low dose of heparin is added to the infusate to prevent clot formation.
Sepsis	Maintain sterile technique when changing dressing, tubing, and solutions; discard infusions hanging >24 hr; avoid using TPN lines for withdrawing blood or giving blood, blood products, or medications. If sepsis is suspected, assist with catheter removal; culture specimens from the catheter tip and exit site; take blood specimen for culture; and administer antibiotics as prescribed.
Catheter occlusion	If solution is infusing sluggishly, flush the line with heparinized saline. If the line is occluded, aspirate clot and contact MD, who may prescribe a thrombolytic agent.

Modified from Roberts PM and Webber KS: Providing nutritional support. In Swearingen PL and Keen JH: Manual of critical care: applying nursing diagnoses to adult critical illness, ed 2, St Louis, Mosby–Year Book, 1991.

Potassium Imbalances

1. **Hyperkalemia** due to excessive enteral or parenteral potassium supplementation or increased tissue catabolism, especially in renal insufficiency. (See Chapter 8.)
2. **Hypokalemia** due to excessive losses from diarrhea or emesis. Hypokalemia also occurs secondary to potassium release and excretion during muscle breakdown in the catabolic patient with normal renal function who is using muscle for energy. (See Chapter 8.)

Calcium Imbalances

1. **Hypercalcemia** due to excessive infusion of calcium or vitamin D. (See Chapter 9.)
2. **Hypocalcemia** due to hypoalbuminemia. Roughly, for every 1 g/dl decrease in serum albumin from 4 g/dl, serum calcium drops 0.8 mg/dl. For example, in a patient with a serum albumin of 3.0 and a serum calcium of 7.5, the corrected calcium value is 8.3 (7.5 + 0.8). An increase in total calories administered or administration of albumin in severe hypoalbuminemia can normalize serum albumin and therefore, serum calcium. (See Chapter 9.)

Phosphorus Imbalances

1. **Hyperphosphatemia** can occur due to an excessive intake of dietary phosphates (e.g., excess dairy products in the renal patient). (See Chapter 10.)
2. **Hypophosphatemia** occurs as a result of transcellular shifts in malnourished tube-fed patients and is associated with high-dose insulin therapy, glucose infusion, diuretics, and diarrhea. (See Chapter 10.)

Magnesium Imbalance

Hypermagnesemia due to increased requirements of magnesium for new tissue synthesis in patients receiving nutritional support. (See Chapter 11.)

References

Alexander JA: Nutrition and translocation, J Parenter Enteral Nutr 14(5):170S–173S, 1990.

Alspach JG: Core curriculum for critical care nursing, ed 4, Philadelphia, 1991, WB Saunders Co.

ASPEN Board of Directors: Guidelines for use of total parenteral nutrition in the hospitalized adult patient, J Parenter Enteral Nutr 10(5):441–445, 1986.

Baas L: Cardiovascular dysfunctions. In Swearingen PL and Keen JH: Manual of critical care: applying nursing diagnoses to adult critical illness, ed 2, St Louis, 1991, Mosby–Year Book.

Berger R and Adams L: Nutritional support in the critical care setting (Part 1), Chest 96(1):139–150, 1986.

Birney MH and Penney DG: Atrial natriuretic peptide: a hormone with implications for clinical practice, Heart Lung 19(2):174–185, 1990.

Blansfield J: Emergency autotransfusion in hypovolemia, Crit Care Nurs Clin North Am 2(2):195–199, 1990.

Bommarito AA, Heinzelmann MJ, and Boysen DA: A new approach to the management of obstructed enteral feeding tubes, Nutrition in Clinical Practice 4:111–114, 1989.

Booth DE and Morris CL: Hyperparathyroidism–the overlooked disorder, J Gerontol Nurs 16(6):16–19, 1990.

Borland C et al: Biochemical and clinical correlates of diuretic therapy in the elderly, Age Ageing 15:357–363, 1986.

Brater DC: Serum electrolyte abnormalities caused by drugs, Prog Drug Res 30:9–69, 1986.

Brenner M and Wellever J: Pulmonary and acid-base assessment, Nurs Clin North Am 25(4):761–770, 1990.

Campbell SM and Kudsk KA: "High tech" metabolic measurements: useful in daily clinical practice? J Parenter Enteral Nutr 12(6):610–612, 1988.

Cogan MG: Atrial natriuretic factor. West J Med 144:591–595, 1986.

Cogan MG: Fluid and electrolytes—physiology and pathophysiology, Norwalk, CT and Los Altos, CA, 1991, Appleton & Lange.

Corbett JV: Laboratory tests and diagnostic procedures with nursing diagnoses, ed 3, Norwalk, CT and Los Altos, CA, 1992, Appleton & Lange.

Cowley AW et al: Osmoregulation during high salt intake: relative importance of drinking and vasopression secretion. Am J Physiol 25:878–886, 1986.

Donner C and Donner, K: The critical difference: pulmonary edema. Am J Nurs 88:59, 1988.

Eisenberg P: Enteral nutrition: indications, formulas, and delivery techniques, Nurs Clin North Am 24(2):315–338, 1989.

Feeney-Stewat F: The sodium bicarbonate controversy, Dimen Crit Care 9(1):22–27, 1990.

Gahart BL: Intravenous medications, ed 7, St Louis, 1991, Mosby–Year Book.

Geheb MA: Clinical approach to the hyperosmolar patient, Crit Care Clinics 5:797–815, 1987.

Goldberger E: A primer of water, electrolyte, and acid-base syndromes, ed 7, Philadelphia, 1986, Lea & Febiger.

Handerhan B: Computing the anion gap, RN 54(7):30–31, 1991.

Hanson-Young M and Whitaker K: High output effluent management, Ostomy/Wound Management 29:30–38, 1990.

Heitz UE: Caring for adults with acid-base imbalances. In Swearingen PL and Keen JH: Manual of critical care: applying nursing diagnoses to adult critical illness, ed 2, St Louis, 1991, Mosby-Year Book.

Hinkle AJ: Pediatric blood and fluid therapy–parts I and II, Cur Rev Nurs Anesth 12(6):41–56, 1989.

Horne MM: Fluid and electrolyte disturbances. In Swearingen PL and Keen JH: Manual of critical care: applying nursing diagnoses to adult critical illness, ed 2, St Louis, 1991, Mosby-Year Book.

Horne MM, Heitz UE, and Swearingen PL: Fluid, electrolyte, and acid-base balance—a case study approach, St Louis, 1991, Mosby-Year Book.

Ichikawa L: Pediatric textbook of fluids and electrolytes, Baltimore, 1990, Williams and Wilkins.

Innerarity SA: Electrolyte emergencies in the critically ill renal patient, Crit Care Nurs Clin North Am 21(1):89–99, 1990.

Janusek L: Metabolic alkalosis: Nursing 90 20(6):52–53, 1990.

Keen JH: Gastrointestinal dysfunctions. In Swearingen PL and Keen JH: Manual of critical care: applying nursing diagnoses to adult critical illness, ed 2, St Louis, 1991, Mosby-Year Book.

Kim MJ, McFarland GK, and McLane AM: Pocket guide to nursing diagnosis, ed 4, St Louis, 1991, Mosby-Year Book.

Kokko JP and Tannen RL: Fluids and electrolytes, ed 2, Philadelphia, 1990, WB Saunders Co.

Kositzke JA: A question of balance—dehydration in the elderly, J Gerontol Nurs 16(5):4–11, 1990.

Koushanpour WK: Renal physiology: principles, structure, and function, ed 2, New York, 1986, Springer-Verlag.

Kresge E: Burns. In Swearingen PL and Keen JH: Manual of critical care: applying nursing diagnoses to adult critical illness, ed 2, St Louis, 1991, Mosby-Year Book.

Lacey JA: Albumin overview: use as a nutritional marker and as a therapeutic intervention, Crit Care Nurse 11(1):46–49, 1991.

Lakshman K and Blackburn GL: Monitoring nutritional status in the critically ill adult, J Clin Monit 2(2):114–120, 1986.

Langer M et al: The prone position in ARDS patients: a clinical study, Chest 94 (1):103–107, 1988.

Lindell K and Wesmiller S: Using arterial blood gases to interpret acid-base balance, Orthop Nurs 8(3):31–34, 1989.

Lipman TH: Assessment of the child with diabetic ketoacidosis, Dimen Crit Care 6(2):82–93, 1987.

Long CL et al: Metabolic response to injury and illness: estimation of energy and protein needs from indirect calorimetry and nitrogen balance, J Parenter Enteral Nutr 3(3):452–456, 1979.

Lorenz A: Lactic acidosis: a nursing challenge, Crit Care 9(4):64–73, 1989.

Lowry SF: Nutrition in the surgical patient. In Schwarz S et al: Principles of surgery, ed 5, New York, 1989, McGraw-Hill Book Co.

Marcuard SP and Stegall KS: Unclogging feeding tubes with pancreatic enzyme, J Parenter Enteral Nutr 14(2):198–200, 1990.

Marcuard SP, Stegall KS, and Trogdon S: Clearing of obstructed feeding tubes, J Parenter Enteral Nutr 13(1):81–83, 1989.

Marik PE et al: Acetazolamide in the treatment of metabolic alkalosis, Heart Lung 20(5):455–459, 1991.

Metheny NA, Spies MA, and Eisenberg P: Measures to test placement of nasoenteral feeding tubes, West J Nurs Res 10(4):367–379, 1988.

Maxwell MH et al: Clinical disorders of fluid and electrolyte metabolism, ed 4, New York, 1987, McGraw-Hill, Inc.

Mims B: Interpreting ABGs, RN 54(3):42–46, 1991.

National Blood Resource Education Program: Transfusion therapy guidelines for nurses, NIH Publication No. 90–2668, 1990.

Needleman P and Greenwald JE: Atriopeptin: a cardiac hormone intimately involved in fluid, electrolyte, and blood pressure homeostasis, New Eng J Med 314:828–834, 1986.

Nicholson LJ: Declogging small-bore feeding tubes, J Parenter Enteral Nutr 11(6):594–597, 1987.

Oster JR: The binge-purge syndrome: a common albeit unappreciated cause of acid-base and fluid-electrolyte disturbances, South Med J 80:58–66, 1987.

Pestana C: Fluids and electrolytes in the surgical patient, ed 4, Baltimore, 1989, Williams and Wilkins.

Pfister S and Bullas J: Arterial blood gas evaluation: metabolic acidemia, Crit Care Nurs 9(1):70–73, 1989.

Phipps W: Medical-surgical nursing, ed 4, St Louis, 1991, Mosby-Year Book.

Rinard G: Water intoxication, Am J Nurs 89(12):1635–1638, 1989.

Roberts PM and Webber KS: Providing nutritional support. In Swearingen PL and Keen JH: Manual of critical care: applying nursing diagnoses to adult critical illness, ed 2, St Louis, 1991, Mosby-Year Book.

Robins EV: Burn shock, Crit Care Nurs Clin North Am 2(2):299–307, 1990.

Rose BD: Clinical physiology of acid-base and electrolyte disorders, ed 3, New York, 1989, McGraw-Hill, Inc.

Russell J: Successful methods for arterial blood gas interpretation, Crit Care Nurs 2(4):14–19, 1991.

Sands JK: Endocrinologic dysfunctions. In Swearingen PL and Keen JH: Manual of critical care: applying nursing diagnoses to adult critical illness, ed 2, St Louis, 1991, Mosby-Year Book.

Schmitz T: The semi-prone position in ARDS: five case studies, Crit Care Nurs 11(5):22–33, 1991.

Schwartz MW: Potassium imbalances, Am J Nurs 87:1292–1299, 1987.

Seldin DW and Giebisch G: The kidney—physiology and pathophysiology, vol 2, New York, 1985, Raven Press.

Shapiro B et al: Clinical application of blood gases, Chicago, 1989, Year Book Medical Publishers.

Smith SL: Postoperative perfusion deficits, Crit Care Nurs Clin North Am 2(4):567–578, 1990.

Steuble BT: Cardiovascular dysfunctions. In Swearingen PL and Keen JH: Manual of critical care: applying nursing diagnoses to adult critical illness, ed 2, St Louis, 1991, Mosby-Year Book.

Stoops CM: Fluid and electrolyte disturbances in the perioperative period, Indiana Medicine 1:13–19, 1987.

Talbot JM: Guidelines for the scientific review of enteral food products for special medical purposes, J Parenter Enteral Nutr 15(3):99S–174S, 1991.

Taylor D: Respiratory alkalosis, Nursing 90 20(7):52–53, 1990.

Thelan LA, Davie JK, and Urden LD: Textbook of critical care nursing: diagnosis and management, St Louis, 1990, Mosby-Year Book.

Thompson JM et al: Mosby's manual of clinical nursing, ed 2, St Louis, 1989, Mosby-Year Book.

Vander AJ: Renal physiology, ed 4, New York, 1991, McGraw-Hill, Inc.

Weiskittel P: Renal-urinary dysfunctions. In Swearingen PL and Keen JH: Manual of critical care: applying nursing diagnoses to adult critical illness, ed 2, St Louis, 1991, Mosby-Year Book.

Yeates S and Blaufuss J: Managing the patient in diabetic ketoacidosis, Focus Crit Care 17(3):240–248, 1990.

Zonszein J: Magnesium and diabetes, Pract Diabetology 10(2):1–5, 1991.

Appendix A: Abbreviations Used in this Manual

ABA: American Burn Association
ABG: Arterial blood gas
ACTH: Adrenocorticotropic hormone
ADH: Antidiuretic hormone
ALS: Amyotropic lateral sclerosis
ANP: Atrial natriuretic peptide
ARDS: Adult respiratory distress syndrome
ARF: Acute renal failure
ATN: Acute tubular necrosis
ATP: Adenosine triphosphate
AV: Atrioventricular
BEE: Basal energy expenditure
BMI: Body mass index
BP: Blood pressure
BSA: Body surface area
BUN: Blood urea nitrogen
Ca^{2+}: Calcium ion
CAVH: Continuous arteriovenous hemofiltration
CBC: Complete blood cell count
CHF: Congestive heart failure
Cl^-: Chloride ion
cm H_2O: Centimeters of water
CNS: Central nervous system
CO: Cardiac output
CO_2: Carbon dioxide
COPD: Chronic obstructive pulmonary disease
CPR: Cardiopulmonary resuscitation

CRF: Chronic renal failure
CVP: Central venous pressure
DCH: Delayed cutaneous hypersensitivity
DDAVP: Desmospressin acetate
DI: Diabetes insipidus
DKA: Diabetic ketoacidosis
dl: Deciliter
DPG: Diphosphoglycerate
ECF: Extracellular fluid
ECV: Effective circulating volume
ECG: Electrocardiogram
FIo$_2$: Fraction of inspired oxygen
GI: Gastrointestinal
H$^+$: Hydrogen ion
H$_2$CO$_3$: Carbonic acid
HCl: Hydrochloric acid
HCO$_3$$^-$: Bicarbonate ion
Hg, Hgb: Hemoglobin
HHNC: Hyperosmolar hyperglycemic nonketotic coma
HOB: Head of bed
HPO$_4$$^{2-}$: Phosphate ion (*also abbreviated* PO$_4$$^{3-}$)
HR: Heart rate
ICF: Intracellular fluid
IM: Intramuscular
I&O: Intake and output
ISF: Interstitial fluid
IU: International unit
Iμ U: International microunit
IV: Intravascular
IVF: Intravascular fluid
K$^+$: Potassium ion
KCl: Potassium chloride
kg: Kilogram
L: Liter
LOC: Level of consciousness
MAP: Mean arterial pressure
mEq: Milliequivalent
mg: Milligram
Mg^{2+}: Magnesium ion
MgSO$_4$: Magnesium sulfate

ml: Milliliter
mm Hg: Millimeters of mercury
mOsm: Milliosmole
N: Nitrogen
Na^+: Sodium ion
NaCl: Sodium chloride
$NaHCO_3$: Sodium bicarbonate
ng: Nanogram
NG: Nasogastric
NH_3: Ammonia
NH_4^+: Ammonium ion
NS: Normal saline, i.e., isotonic solution of NaCl
O_2: Oxygen
OTC: Over-the-counter
P: Phosphorus
PA: Pulmonary artery
Pa_{CO_2}: Carbon dioxide tension of arterial blood
Pa_{O_2}: Oxygen tension of arterial blood
PAP: Pulmonary artery pressure
PAWP: Pulmonary artery wedge pressure
pg: Picogram
PO_4^{3-}: Phosphate ion (*also abbreviated* HPO_4^{2-})
PRBCs: Packed red blood cells
prn: As needed
PTH: Parathyroid hormone
PVC: Premature ventricular contractions
q: Every
RBC: Red blood cell
RDA: Recommended daily allowance
ROM: Range of motion
RR: Respiratory rate
RTA: Renal tubular acidosis
SC: Subcutaneous
SIADH: Syndrome of inappropriate antidiuretic hormone
SOB: Shortness of breath
stat: Immediately
SVR: Systemic vascular resistance
TBW: Total body water
TCF: Transcellular fluid
TKO: To keep open

TPN: Total parenteral nutrition
μg: Microgram
μ IU: Microinternational unit
VS: Vital sign
WBC: White blood cell
WOB: Work of breathing

Appendix B: Glossary

Acidemia: Change of pH in arterial blood to <7.40.

Acidosis: Abnormal accumulation of acid or loss of base from the body.

Acids: Substances that can give up a hydrogen ion.

Active transport: The movement of solutes across a cell membrane in the absence of a favorable electrochemical or concentration gradient; requires energy.

Acute renal failure (ARF): A sudden loss of renal function that is usually reversible.

Aldosterone: A mineralocorticoid hormone released by the adrenal cortex that increases the reabsorption (saving) of sodium and secretion and excretion of potassium and hydrogen by the kidneys.

Alkalemia: Increase in arterial pH to >7.40.

Alkalosis: Abnormal accumulation of bicarbonate or loss of acid in the body.

Anaerobic metabolism: Occurs when there is not enough oxygen available for metabolism and alternate pathways are used, resulting in an accumulation of organic acids (lactic acidosis).

Analog: A substance with structure and function similar to another substance.

Anasarca: Severe generalized edema.

Angiotensin: A polypeptide found in the blood and formed by the action of renin on the α-2-globulin, angiotensinogen. *Angiotensin I* is converted to *angiotensin II*. Angiotensin II, a potent vasoconstrictor, acts on the adrenal cortex to stimulate the release of aldosterone.

Anions: Ions that develop a negative charge in solution. Examples of the body's most common anions include chloride ion, bicarbonate ion, and phosphate ion. Proteins are another important group of anions.

Anion gap: Reflection of the anions in plasma (e.g., phosphates, sulfates, and proteinates) that normally are unmeasured. Anion gap is helpful in the differential diagnosis of metabolic acidosis or mixed acid-base disorders.

Antidiuretic hormone (ADH): Produced by the hypothalamus and released by the posterior pituitary gland, it increases reabsorption (saving) of water by the kidneys, allowing excretion of a concentrated urine. In addition, ADH is an arterial vasoconstrictor that increases blood pressure by increasing vascular resistance.

Anuria: The production of ≤100 ml of urine in 24 hours.

Arterial blood gases (ABGs): Measurement of pH, carbon dioxide tension, and oxygen tension of arterial blood to evaluate acid-base and pulmonary functions.

Asterixis: Hand-flapping tremor that occurs with extension of the arm and dorsiflexion of the wrist. It is often seen with metabolic disorders.

Atrial natriuretic factor (ANF): Another term for atrial natriuretic peptide.

Atrial natriuretic peptide (ANP): Recently identified hormone that is released by the cardiac atria in response to an increased vascular volume. ANP reduces blood pressure and vascular volume.

Azotemia: Increased retention of metabolic wastes.

Baroreceptors: Pressure-sensitive nerve endings located in the carotid sinuses, aortic arch, cardiac atria, and renal vessels, which respond to changes in blood pressure *via* changes in stretch in the arterial wall, leading to changes in cardiac output, vascular resistance, thirst, and renal handling of sodium and water.

Bases: Substances that can take on a hydrogen ion.

Bicarbonate: The body's most important and abundant buffer. It is generated in the kidney and aids in excretion of hydrogen ion.

Buffers: Substances that combine with excess acid or base, resulting in a minimally altered pH.

Capillary membrane: Separates the intravascular fluid from the interstitial fluid.

Cardiac output (CO): Product of heart rate times stroke volume (i.e., the amount of blood moved with each contraction of the left ventricle/min). Normal value is 4-7 L/min for the adult.

Cations: Ions that develop a positive charge in solution and are attracted to negative electrons. Examples of the body's most common cations include sodium ions, potassium ions, calcium ions, magnesium ions, and hydrogen ions.

Cell membrane: Composed of lipids and protein, this membrane separates intracellular fluid from the interstitial fluid.

Central venous pressure (CVP): Measurement of the right atrial pressure and right ventricular end-diastolic pressure *via* a catheter inserted in or near the right atrium.

Chronic renal failure (CRF): An irreversible loss of kidney function, also known as *end-stage renal disease.*

Chvostek's sign: A signal of tetany occurring with hypocalcemia or hypomagnesemia, it is considered positive when there is unilateral contraction of the facial and eyelid muscles in response to facial nerve percussion.

Colloid: In the medical vernacular, colloid is an IV fluid that contains solutes *that do not readily* cross the capillary membrane. Dextran, blood, albumin, mannitol, and plasma are all colloids. When combined with water, colloids do not form true solutions.

Concentration gradient: The concentration difference between an area of a high concentration and an area of low concentration of the same substance.

Crystalloid: In the medical vernacular, crystalloid is an IV fluid that contains solutes *that readily* cross the capillary membrane. Examples include dextrose or electrolyte solutions. When combined with water, crystalloids dissolve and form true solutions.

Diffusion: Random movement of particles through a solution or gas, in which the particles move from an area of high concentration to an area of low concentration. When diffusion of a particular solute is dependent on the availability of a carrier substance, it is termed *facilitated* diffusion. Diffusion not dependent on a carrier substance is termed *simple* diffusion.

Edema: Palpable swelling of the interstitial space that can be either localized or generalized.

Effective circulating volume (ECV): The portion of intravascular volume that actually perfuses the tissues. For example, in congestive heart failure intravascular volume increases because of sodium and water retention, yet ECV decreases because of the pooling of blood in the venous circuit.

Effective osmolality: Changes in osmolality that will cause water to move from one compartment to another. If a substance has an equal concentration on both sides of the membrane, there is no effective osmolality. *Tonicity* is another term for effective osmolality.

Electrolytes: Substances (solutes) that dissociate in solution and conduct an electrical current. Electrolytes dissociate into positive ions (cations) and negative ions (anions).

Epithelial membrane: Separates interstitial fluid and intravascular fluid from the transcellular fluid and produces transcellular fluid.

Erythropoietin: A glycoprotein hormone released by the renal cells in response to low oxygen levels, which stimulates production of red blood cells by the bone marrow.

Extracellular fluid (ECF): Fluid found outside the cells, comprising approximately one third of the body's fluid (in the adult).

Filtration: Movement of water and solutes from an area of high hydraulic pressure to an area of low hydraulic pressure.

Glomerular filtration rate (GFR): The volume of fluid crossing the glomerular membrane each minute.

Hemolysis: Breakdown of red blood cells that may occur if blood is exposed to a hypotonic solution.

Homeostasis: Physiologic balance in which there is relative constancy in the body's environment, maintained by adaptive responses.

Hydrostatic pressure: Pressure created by the weight of fluid.

Hydraulic pressure: One of the factors that affects the movement of fluid across the capillary membrane. It is a combination of hydrostatic pressure and the pressure created by the pump action of the heart. The terms *hydrostatic pressure* and *hydraulic pressure* are often used interchangeably.

Hypercapnia: Increased amounts of carbon dioxide in the blood caused by hypoventilation. It is also known as hypercarbia.

Hypertonicity: State in which a solution's effective osmolality is greater than that of the body's fluids.

Hyperventilation: Any process resulting in a decreased Pa_{CO_2}.

Hypervolemia: Expansion of the extracellular fluid volume. Usually used to describe the expansion of the intravascular portion of the extracellular fluid.

Hypocapnia: Decreased amounts of carbon dioxide in the blood caused by hyperventilation. It is also known as hypocarbia.

Hypotonicity: State in which a solution's effective osmolality is greater than that of the body's fluids.

Hypoventilation: Any process resulting in an increased $Paco_2$.

Hypovolemia: A reduction in the extracellular fluid volume. Usually used to describe a reduction in the volume of the intravascular portion of the extracellular fluid.

Insensible fluid: Imperceptible loss of fluid through the skin or respiratory system *via* evaporation. Because it is nearly free of electrolytes, insensible fluid loss is considered pure water loss.

Interstitial fluid (ISF): The fluid surrounding the cells, including lymph fluid.

Intracellular fluid (ICF): Fluid contained within the cells, comprising approximately two thirds of the body's fluid (in the adult).

Intravascular fluid (IVF): Fluid contained within the blood vessels (i.e., plasma).

Isohydric principle: This principle states that a change in the hydrogen ion concentration will affect the ratio of acids to bases in all buffer systems.

Isotonic solutions: Fluids with the same effective osmolality as body fluids.

Kussmaul respirations: Rapid, deep, *sighing* breaths.

Mean arterial pressure (MAP): A reflection of the average pressure within the arterial tree throughout the cardiac cycle. The normal value is 70-105 mm Hg.

Metastatic calcifications: Precipitation and deposition of calcium phosphate in the soft tissue, joints, and arteries, also known as soft tissue calcifications.

Milk-alkali syndrome: Renal dysfunction and metabolic alkalosis resulting from chronic ingestion of excessive amounts of absorbable alkali (i.e., milk and calcium carbonate).

Minute ventilation: Respiratory rate × tidal volume.

Nonelectrolytes: Substances that do not dissociate (separate) in solution. Examples include glucose, urea, creatinine, and bilirubin.

Nonvolatile (fixed) acid: Any acid that cannot be vaporized and excreted by the lungs.

Oliguria: Urinary output of <400 ml/24 hr.

Oncotic pressure: Osmotic pressure exerted by protein.

Osmolality: The number of particles contained in body fluids, i.e., concentration; measured in mOsm/kg of water.

Osmolarity: Like osmolality, it is a term used to describe the concentration of fluids; measured in mOsm/L of solution.

Osmosis: Movement of water across a semipermeable membrane from an area of lower solute concentration to an area of higher solute concentration.

Osmotic diuresis: Increased urine output caused by such substances as mannitol, glucose, or contrast media, which are excreted in the urine and reduce water reabsorption.

Osmotic pressure: The pressure that *pulls* water across a semipermeable membrane when the membrane separates two solutions with different concentrations. See *osmosis*.

Oxygen saturation: The degree to which hemoglobin is combined with oxygen.

pH: Measurement of hydrogen ion concentration in body fluids reflecting one of the following states: normal (7.40), acidic (<7.40), or alkalotic (>7.40).

Plasma: The fluid portion of the blood containing water, protein, and electrolytes.

Polyuria: Excessive urine output.

Pulmonary artery pressure (PAP): Pressure measured in the pulmonary artery. When pulmonary function is normal, it reflects the pressure within the left ventricle at the end of diastole. PAP is used to evaluate left ventricular function and fluid volume. Normal PAP is 20 to 30/8 to 15 mm Hg.

Pulmonary artery wedge pressure (PAWP): Measurement of the pulmonary capillary pressure by means of a balloon-tipped catheter passed into the distal pulmonary artery. It provides a more accurate reflection of left ventricular end-diastolic pressure than pulmonary artery pressure. Normal PAWP is 6-12 mm Hg.

Renin: Proteolytic enzyme produced and released by specialized cells located in the arterioles of the kidney. Renin is released in response to decreased renal perfusion or stimulation of the sympathetic nervous system and is important in the formation of angiotensin.

Sensible fluid: Perceptible loss of body fluid (i.e., sweat) *via* the skin; contains a significant amount of electrolytes.

Serum: Plasma minus the fibrinogen and other clotting factors;

i.e., the fluid that remains after a blood specimen has been allowed to form a clot.

Sodium-potassium pump: A physiologic mechanism present in all body cell membranes that transports sodium from the inside of the cell to the outside and transports potassium from the outside of the cell to the inside. It requires energy and the presence of adequate magnesium.

Solutes: Dissolved particles found in body fluids. There are two types: electrolytes and nonelectrolytes.

Specific gravity: Measurement of the weight of a substance in relationship to water. Water = 1.000.

Substrate: A substance that is acted upon (and changed by) an enzyme during a chemical reaction.

Syndrome of inappropriate antidiuretic hormone (SIADH): A condition in which there is inappropriate hypothalamic production or enhanced action or ectopic production of antidiuretic hormone resulting in excess water retention.

Systemic vascular resistance (SVR): Clinical measurement of the resistance in vessels, which is used to determine workload of the left ventricle (afterload). Normal SVR is 900-1200 dynes/sec/cm^{-5}.

Tachypnea: Increased respiratory rate. It is also called *hyperpnea*.

Third-space fluid shift: The loss of extracellular fluid into a normally nonequilibrating space. Although the fluid has not been lost from the body, it is temporarily unavailable to the intracellular fluid or extracellular fluid for its use.

Tidal volume: Normal resting volume of ventilation.

Tonicity: Another term for *effective osmolality*.

Transcellular fluid (TCF): Fluid secreted by epithelial cells. These fluids include cerebrospinal, pericardial, pleural, synovial, and intraocular fluids and digestive secretions.

Trousseau's sign: Ischemia-induced carpal spasm that occurs with hypocalcemia and hypomagnesemia. It may be elicited by applying a blood pressure cuff to the upper arm and inflating it past systolic blood pressure for 2 minutes.

Ventilation-perfusion mismatch: An inequality in the ratio between ventilation and perfusion that occurs with shunting of venous blood past unventilated alveoli.

Volatile acid: An acid that can be vaporized and eliminated by the lungs (i.e., carbon dioxide).

Appendix C: Effects of Age on Fluid, Electrolyte, and Acid-Base Balance

Infants and Children

- Relative to their size, infants and children have a greater body surface area (BSA) (both external and internal) than the adult, and thus have a greater potential for fluid loss *via* the skin and gastrointestinal tract.
- Infants and children have a higher percentage of total body water (TBW) than adults. The greater percentage of the infant's body water is extracellular. As cellular growth occurs, more fluid becomes intracellular.
- Infants have a decreased ability to concentrate their urine, whereas at the same time they have an increased solute load to excrete because of their increased caloric need. These two factors result in a relatively greater obligatory fluid loss, meaning that they must produce a relatively larger volume of urine in order to excrete their daily load of metabolic wastes.
- The daily intake and output (I&O) for infants (e.g., 650 ml) is equal to approximately half the volume of their extracellular fluid (ECF) (e.g., 1300 ml), as compared to adults, whose daily I&O (e.g., 2500 ml) is approximately one sixth of their ECF (e.g., 15.0 L). Thus infants can lose a volume equal to their ECF in 2 days, whereas it takes an adult 6 days to do the same.

- Because of an infant's small size and decreased ability to excrete excess fluid, IV fluid administration necessitates caution *via* use of monitored pumps.
- Infants are less able to compensate for acidosis because of their decreased ability to acidify urine.
- Infants are at increased risk for developing hypernatremia since they are unable to verbalize thirst. Remember that thirst is the body's primary defense against symptomatic hypernatremia.
- Children have an increased incidence and intensity of fever, upper respiratory infections, and gastroenteritis, which can lead to abnormal fluid and electrolyte loss. See Chapter 18 for a discussion of the various fluid and electrolyte imbalances that occur with loss of upper and lower gastrointestinal contents.
- Infants and small children are prone to fluid volume deficit caused by a combination of the factors listed previously. Unfortunately, some of the common indicators of fluid volume deficit are less reliable in the infant or small child. Infants are unable to verbalize thirst, although their cries may become increasingly high-pitched. Skin turgor also may be a less reliable sign. Skin turgor may appear normal in the obese infant because of increased subcutaneous fat, or it may appear abnormal in the adequately hydrated but undernourished infant. Irritability is an early indicator of hypovolemia. Sunken fontanels, a traditional indicator of dehydration, does not occur until there has been moderate to severe fluid loss.

The Older Adult

- Weight (body fat) tends to increase with advancing age, thus the percentage of TBW decreases. Recall that fat cells contain little water. The percentage of TBW increases in the emaciated individual who has lost significant body fat.
- Renal function decreases with advancing age. Glomerular filtration rate drops; thus the older adult is less likely to compensate for an increased metabolic load. There is also a reduction in the ability to concentrate urine, resulting in greater obligatory water losses. The older adult must pro-

duce a larger volume of urine to excrete the same amount of metabolic waste as the younger adult.

- In the older adult, the kidneys are less able to compensate for an acid load, owing to decreased formation of ammonia. (Ammonia produced by the renal tubular cell diffuses into the lumen of the tubule and combines with hydrogen to form ammonium, which is then excreted in the urine. In this way, ammonia acts as a urinary buffer, allowing increased excretion of hydrogen ions.) Normally, ammonia production increases in the presence of an acid load.

- Decreased respiratory function also reduces the older adult's ability to compensate for acid-base imbalance. The older adult is also more likely to develop hypoxemia.

- There is a reduction in the secretion of HCl by the stomach, which may affect the individual's ability to tolerate certain foods. The older adult is especially prone to constipation because of decreased gastrointestinal tract motility. Limited fluid intake, a restricted diet, and a reduced level of physical activity may contribute to the development of constipation. Excessive or inappropriate use of laxatives may lead to problems with diarrhea.

- As the skin ages, there is a reduction in insensible and sensible water loss secondary to decreased skin hydration and decreased functioning of the sweat glands. Thus the skin is less efficient in cooling the body, and the skin tends to be dry. In addition, skin turgor is a less reliable indicator of fluid status due to decreased skin elasticity.

- Older adults are at increased risk for developing hypernatremia because they have a less sensitive thirst center and may have problems with obtaining fluids (e.g., impaired mobility) or expressing their desire for fluids (e.g., the individual who has suffered a stroke). Thirst is the body's primary defense against symptomatic hypernatremia.

Appendix D: Laboratory Tests Discussed in this Manual (Normal Values)*

Complete Blood Count (CBC)	Adult Normal Values
Hemoglobin	Male: 14-18 g/dl
	Female: 12-16 g/dl
Hematocrit	Male: 40%-54%
	Female: 37%-47%
Red blood cell (RBC) count	Male: 4.5-6.0 million/μl
	Female: 4.0-5.5 million/μl
White blood cell (WBC) count	4500-11,000/μl
Neutrophils	54%-75% (3000-7500/μl)
Band neutrophils	3%-8% (150-700μl)
Lymphocytes	25%-40% (1500-4500/μl)
Monocytes	2%-8% (100-500/μl)
Eosinophils	1%-4% (50-400/μl)
Basophils	0%-1% (25-100/μl)
Platelet count	150,000-400,000/μl

*Normal values may vary significantly with different laboratory methods of testing.

Serum, Plasma, and Whole Blood Chemistry	Normal Values
ACTH	8 AM-10 AM <100 pg/ml
ADH	0-2 pg/ml/serum osmolality <285 mOsm/kg; 2-12 pg/ml/serum osmolality >290 mOsm/kg
Albumin	3.5-5.5 g/dl
Aldosterone	Male: 6-22 ng/dl Female: 4-31 ng/dl
Ammonia	Adult: 15–110 μg/dl Child: 56–80 μg/dl Newborn: 90–150 μg/dl
Amylase	60-180 Somogyi U/dl
Base, total	145-160 mEq/L
Bicarbonate	22-26 mEq/L
Bilirubin	Total: 0.3-1.4 mg/dl
ABGs	
pH	7.35-7.45
$Paco_2$	35-45 mm Hg
Pao_2	80-95 mm Hg
O_2 saturation	95%-99%
Blood urea nitrogen	6–20 mg/dl
Calcitonin	<100 pg/ml
Calcium	8.5-10.5 mg/dl; 4.3-5.3 mEq/L
Chloride	95-108 mEq/L
Cortisol	8 AM-10 AM: 5-25 μg/dl 4 PM-12 AM (midnight): 2-18 μg/dl
CO_2 content (Total CO_2)	22-28 mEq/L
CPK	Male: 55-170 U/L Female: 30-135 U/L
Creatinine	0.6-1.5 mg/dl
Creatinine clearance	Male: 107-141 ml/min Female: 87-132 ml/min
Globulins, total	1.5-3.5 g/dl

ACTH = adrenocorticotropic hormone; ADH = antidiuretic hormone; ABGs = arterial blood gases; $Paco_2$ = carbon dioxide tension of arterial blood; Pao_2 = oxygen tension of arterial blood; O_2 = oxygen; CO_2 = carbon dioxide; CPK = creatinine phosphokinase.

Serum, Plasma, and Whole Blood Chemistry	Normal Values
Glucose, fasting	True glucose: 65-110 mg/dl
	All sugars: 80-120 mg/dl
Glucose, 2-hr postprandial	<145 mg/dl
Glucose tolerance	Fasting: 65-110 mg/dl
Intravenous	5 min: maximum 250 mg/dl
	60 min: decrease
	2 hr: <120 mg/dl
	3 hr: 65-110 mg/dl
Oral	Fasting: 65-110 mg/dl
	30 min: <155 mg/dl
	1 hr: <165 mg/dl
	2 hr: <120 mg/dl
	3 hr: ≤65-110 mg/dl
17-OCHS	Male: 7-19 µg/dl
	Female: 9-21 µg/dl
Insulin	11-240 µIU/ml
	4-24 µU/ml
Iron	Total: 60-200 µg/dl
	Male, average: 125 µg/dl
	Female, average: 100 µg/dl
	Elderly: 60-80 µg/dl
Ketone bodies	2-4 µg/dl
Lactic acid	Arterial: 0.5-1.6 mEq/L
	Venous: 1.5-2.2 mEq/L
Magnesium	1.8-3.0 mg/dl
	1.5-2.5 mEq/L
Osmolality	280-300 mOsm/kg
Parathyroid hormone	<2000 pg/ml
Phosphatase, acid	0-1.1 U/ml (Bodansky)
	1-4 U/ml (King-Armstrong)
	0.13-0.63 U/ml (Bessey-Lowery)
Phosphatase alkaline	1.5-4.5 U/dl (Bodansky)
	4-13 U/dl (King-Armstrong)
	0.8-2.3 U/ml (Bessey-Lowery)
Phosphorus	2.5-4.5 mg/dl; 1.7-2.6 mEq/L
Potassium	3.5-5.0 mEq/L

Serum, Plasma, and Whole Blood Chemistry	Normal Values
Renin	Normal sodium intake
	Supine (4-6 hr): 0.5-1.6 ng/ml/hr
	Sitting (4 hr): 1.8-3.6 ng/ml/hr
	Low sodium intake
	Supine (4-6 hr): 2.2-4.4 ng/ml/hr
	Sitting (4 hr): 4.0-8.1 ng/ml/hr
Sodium	137-147 mEq/L
Thyroid stimulating hormone (TSH)	4.6 μU/ml
Urea clearance Serum/ 24-hr urine	64-99 ml/min (maximum clearance)
	41-65 ml/min (standard clearance)
Uric acid	Male: 2.1-7.5 mg/dl
	Female: 2.0-6.6 mg/dl

Urine Chemistry	Normal Values
Albumin	
Random	Negative
24-hr	10-100 mg/24 hr
Amylase	
2-hr	35-260 (Somogyi) U/hr
24-hr	80-5000 U/24 hr
Bilirubin	
Random	Negative: 0.02 mg/dl
Calcium	
Random	1+ turbidity; 10 mg/dl
24-hr	50-300 mg/24 hr
Creatinine	
24-hr	Male: 20-26 mg/kg/24 hr
	Female: 14-22 mg/kg/24 hr
Creatinine clearance	Male: 107-141 ml/min
	Female: 87-132 ml/min

Urine Chemistry	Normal Values
Glucose	
Random	Negative: 15 mg/dl
24-hr	130 mg/24 hr
Ketone	
24-hr	Negative: 0.3-2.0 mg/dl
Osmolality	
Random	350-700 mOsm/kg
24-hr	300-900 mOsm/kg
Physiologic range	50-1400 mOsm/kg
pH	
Random	4.6-8.0
Phosphorus	
24-hr	0.9-1.3 g; 0.2-0.6 mEq/L
Protein	
Random	Negative: 2-8 mg/dl
24-hr	40-150 mg
Sodium	
Random	50-130 mEq/L
24-hr	40-220 mEq/L
Specific gravity	
Random	1.010-1.020
After fluid restriction	1.025-1.035
Sugar	
Random	Negative
Urea clearance	
24-hr	64-99 ml/min (maximum)
	41-65 ml/min (standard)
Urea nitrogen	
24-hr	6-17 g

Index

Gentamicin—cont'd
  in renal failure, 223
Glomerulonephritis
  acute, in renal failure, 222
  and chronic renal failure, 222
Glucocorticoid deficiency, and adrenal
      insufficiency, 213-214
Glucose, 6, 9-10, 12
  for hyperkalemia, 105
Glucosuria, 11
Guanethidine, in renal failure, 223

H

Halothane, and hepatic failure, 230
Hands, assessment of veins in, 34
Harris and Benedict equations of basal
      energy expenditure, 245
HCO_3, in arterial blood analysis, 150
Heart rate, 32
Hematocrit, 38
  in hypovolemia, 54, 69
Hemodialysis
  in hypercalcemia, 115
  for metabolic acidosis, 173
Hemodynamic monitoring, 29, 31
  for hyponatremia, 90-91
Hemolytic reaction, acute, 82-83
Hepatic, chronic insufficiency, and
      respiratory alkalosis, 166
Hepatic cirrhosis, edema in, 75
Hepatic encephalopathy, and total
      parenteral nutrition, 257
Hepatic failure, 229-230
  and nutritional support, 247
  potential fluid, electrolyte, and
      acid-base disturbances,
      230-231
Hepatorenal syndrome
  acute, in renal failure, 222
  and hepatic failure, 229
Hetastarch, 65
Hip, fractured, and third-space shift,
      52
Homeostasis, 23
Hydrochloric acid (HCl), 191
  in metabolic alkalosis, 178
Hydrochlorothiazide, and hepatic
      failure, 230
Hydrocortisone, 199
Hydro-duiril. *See* Thiazides
Hydrostatic pressure, 10
Hygrotin. *See* Chlorothalidone
Hyperactive reflexes, 35
Hyperadrenocorticism, in metabolic
      alkalosis, 179-180, 181

Hyperaldosteronism
  in hypokalemia, 98
  in hypomagnesemia, 132
Hypercalcemia
  and acute pancreatitis, 227
  assessment, 114
  collaborative management, 115
  diagnostic tests, 114-115
  nursing diagnoses and interventions,
      115-117
  and nutritional support, 260
  patient-family teaching guidelines,
      117
Hypercapnia, chronic, 158
Hyperglycemia, 11, 13
  as cause of pseudohyponatremia, 51
  and hyperosmolar hyperglycemic
      nonketotic coma, 203-204
  and hyperosmolarity, 201
  and serum osmolarity, 38
Hyperkalemia, 103-104
  and acute adrenal insufficiency, 214
  assessment, 54, 104
  in burns, 239
  collaborative management, 105-106
  and diabetic ketoacidosis, 202
  diagnostic tests, 104-105
  and diuretic therapy, 77
  and hepatic failure, 231
  nursing diagnoses and interventions,
      106-107
  and nutritional support, 260
  patient-family teaching guidelines,
      107
  and renal failure, 225
  and surgical disturbances, 200
Hyperlipidemia, as cause of
      pseudohyponatremia, 51
Hypermagnesemia, 136
  assessment, 136-137
  collaborative management, 137
  diagnostic tests, 137
  nursing diagnoses and interventions,
      137-139
  and nutritional support, 260
  patient-family teaching guidelines,
      139
  and renal failure, 225
Hypermetabolic states, and respiratory
      alkalosis, 164
Hypernatremia, 93
  and aging, 279
  assessment, 55, 93-94
  collaborative management, 94-95
  and diabetes insipidus, 212
  and diabetic ketoacidosis, 202